AIoT Innovations in Digital Health

Artificial Intelligence (AI) innovations in digital health offer unprecedented opportunities to facilitate human health and provide tools and techniques that reduce overall costs. This book discusses the use of AI to improve diagnostic accuracy, patient monitoring, the use of remote diagnostic tools, identification of life-threatening diseases, medical robotics applications, drug discovery, technology-driven solutions, and much more.

AIoT Innovations in Digital Health: Emerging Trends, Challenges, and Solutions presents integrated technologies such as Green Computing, IoT, and Big Data using AI, Machine Learning, Deep Learning, and Federated Learning for Healthcare. It discusses the future of medical robotics using Machine Learning and highlights the use of Federated Learning-based patient monitoring applications. This book also elaborates on the role that AI and Machine Learning play in drug discovery.

Interested readers will include anyone working in or involved in smart healthcare research, which includes, but is not limited to, healthcare specialists, computer science engineers, electronics engineers, systems engineers, and pharmaceutical practitioners.

Artificial Intelligence in Smart Healthcare Systems

Series Editors:
Vishal Jain and Jyotir Moy Chatterjee

The progress of the healthcare sector is incremental as it learns from associations between data over time through the application of suitable big data and IoT frameworks and patterns. Many healthcare service providers are employing IoT-enabled devices for monitoring patient health care, but their diagnoses and prescriptions are instance-specific only. However, these IoT-enabled healthcare devices are generating volumes of data (Big-IoT Data) that can be analyzed for more accurate diagnosis and prescriptions. A major challenge in the above realm is the effective and accurate learning of unstructured clinical data through the application of precise algorithms. Incorrect input data leading to erroneous outputs with false positives shall be intolerable in healthcare as patient's lives are at stake. This new book series addresses various aspects of how smart healthcare can be used to detect and analyze diseases, the underlying methodologies, and related security concerns. Healthcare is a multidisciplinary field that involves a range of factors like the financial system, social factors, health technologies, and organizational structures that affect the healthcare provided to individuals, families, institutions, organizations, and populations. The goals of healthcare services include patient safety, timeliness, effectiveness, efficiency, and equity. Smart healthcare consists of m-health, e-health, electronic resource management, smart and intelligent home services, and medical devices. The Internet of Things (IoT) is a system comprising real-world things that interact and communicate with each other via networking technologies. The wide range of potential applications of IoT includes healthcare services. IoT-enabled healthcare technologies are suitable for remote health monitoring, including rehabilitation, assisted ambient living, etc. In turn, healthcare analytics can be applied to the data gathered from different areas to improve healthcare at a minimum expense.

This new book series is designed to be a first-choice reference at university libraries, academic institutions, research and development centers, information technology centers, and any institutions interested in using, designing, modeling, and analyzing intelligent healthcare services. Successful application of deep learning frameworks to enable meaningful, cost-effective personalized healthcare services is the primary aim of the healthcare industry in the present scenario. However, realizing this goal requires effective understanding, application, and amalgamation of IoT, Big Data, and several other computing technologies to deploy such systems in an effective manner. This series shall help clarify the understanding of certain key mechanisms and technologies helpful in realizing such systems.

AIoT Innovations in Digital Health: Emerging Trends, Challenges, and Solutions
Edited by Inam Ullah, Salma El Hajjami, Shashi Kant Gupta, Hameedur Rahman, Thiagarajan Yogamoorthi, Inam Ullah, and Muhammad Adnan Khan

For more information about this series, please visit Artificial Intelligence in Smart Healthcare Systems – Book Series – Routledge & CRC Press.

AIoT Innovations in Digital Health

Emerging Trends, Challenges, and Solutions

Edited by
Inam Ullah Khan, Salma El Hajjami,
Shashi Kant Gupta, Hameedur Rahman,
Thiagarajan Yogamoorthi, Inam Ullah,
and Muhammad Adnan Khan

CRC Press
Taylor & Francis Group
Boca Raton London New York

CRC Press is an imprint of the
Taylor & Francis Group, an **informa** business

Cover image: Getty Images

First edition published 2025
by CRC Press
2385 NW Executive Center Drive, Suite 320, Boca Raton FL 33431

and by CRC Press
4 Park Square, Milton Park, Abingdon, Oxon, OX14 4RN

CRC Press is an imprint of Taylor & Francis Group, LLC

ISBN: 978-1-032-74441-4 (hbk)
ISBN: 978-1-032-74570-1 (pbk)
ISBN: 978-1-003-46989-6 (ebk)

DOI: 10.1201/9781003469896

Typeset in Times
by codeMantra

Contents

Preface

AIoT Innovations in Digital Health: Emerging Trends, Challenges, and Solutions explores the transformative impact of Artificial Intelligence and the Internet of Things on the field of digital health. In an era where technology and healthcare are increasingly intertwined, this book serves as a crucial resource for understanding the latest advancements and emerging trends that are reshaping how we approach medical diagnostics, treatment, and patient management. Each chapter provides in-depth insights into a range of topics, from leveraging deep learning for sentiment analysis of healthcare-related social media to employing sophisticated hybrid algorithms and AI techniques for predicting and diagnosing complex health conditions such as heart disease, lung cancer, and brain tumors. The volume also addresses critical issues related to privacy and security in AIoT applications, offering a balanced view of the challenges and solutions necessary for safeguarding sensitive health data. Furthermore, it explores innovative IoT-assisted solutions for chronic disease management and the integration of AI in plant science for improved agricultural outcomes. By bringing together leading experts and researchers, this book aims to foster a deeper understanding of how AIoT innovations are driving progress in digital health while navigating the associated hurdles. It is our hope that this collection will not only inform but also inspire continued research, collaboration, and development in this rapidly evolving field, ultimately contributing to more effective and equitable healthcare solutions worldwide.

Chapter 1 delves into leveraging deep learning techniques to analyze the sentiment of user tweets, focusing on detecting polarity in opinions related to healthcare services. It explores how sentiment analysis can aid in understanding public perceptions and improving healthcare delivery.

Chapter 2 introduces a novel hybrid approach combining a Non-Sorted Genetic Algorithm with Logistic Regression to enhance the prediction accuracy for heart diseases. It discusses how this integrated method improves diagnostic precision and supports effective risk assessment.

Chapter 3 presents a cutting-edge hybrid blockchain mechanism designed for IoT-based healthcare systems to detect the recurrence of blood cancer. It highlights how blockchain technology ensures data integrity and enhances the reliability of cancer monitoring applications.

Chapter 4 discusses a comprehensive IoT-assisted solution aimed at managing chronic kidney disease more effectively. It evaluates how integrating IoT technology can facilitate continuous monitoring and personalized treatment plans for patients.

Chapter 5 addresses the critical privacy and security concerns associated with AI and IoT in the healthcare industry. It reviews various methods, tools, and applications while identifying key open challenges and proposing potential solutions.

Chapter 6 focuses on the development of an ontology-based expert system designed to aid in the diagnosis of lung cancer. It explores how ontological frameworks can enhance diagnostic accuracy and support clinical decision-making.

Chapter 7 examines the application of AI in conjunction with IoT technologies for the detection of brain tumors in MRI images. It highlights the advancements in image analysis and the potential for improved diagnostic outcomes.

Chapter 8 provides insights into the use of advanced AI techniques for detecting breast cancer and assessing its severity through image analysis. It discusses the impact of these technologies on early diagnosis and treatment planning.

Chapter 9 explores a cognitive machine learning-based system designed to detect intrusions related to life-threatening diseases. It emphasizes how this system enhances disease surveillance and early intervention through sophisticated learning algorithms.

About the Editors

Dr. Inam Ullah Khan is the Founder of AI-Explain Your Science (AI-EYS) and a Senior Member of IEEE. He is also a member of the International Association of Engineers (IAENG), IEEE Young Professionals, IEEE Systems Council, IAENG Society of Artificial Intelligence, IAENG Society of Computer Science, IAENG Society of Internet Computing and Web Services, IAENG Society of Information System Engineering, IAENG Society of Scientific Computing, IAENG Society of Software Engineering, and IAENG Society of Wireless Networks. He is a Mentor of Artificial Intelligence at Corvit Systems, Rawalpindi, Pakistan, and works remotely as a Global Mentor/Guest Lecturer at Impact Xcelerator, School of Science & Technology, IE University, Madrid, Spain. Currently, he also serves as a Trainer at the National Vocational and Technical Training Commission (NVTTC) in Pakistan. Previously, he was a Visiting Researcher at King's College London, UK, and has been a faculty member at several universities in Pakistan, including the National University of Technology, Islamabad; Center for Emerging Sciences, Engineering & Technology (CESET), Islamabad; Abdul Wali Khan University (Garden Campus, Timergara Campus); University of Swat; and Shaheed Zulfikar Ali Bhutto Institute of Science and Technology (SZABIST), Islamabad Campus. He earned his Ph.D. in Electronics Engineering from the Department of Electronic Engineering at Isra University, Islamabad Campus, School of Engineering & Applied Sciences (SEAS). He also holds an M.S. in Electronic Engineering from the same institution and completed his undergraduate degree in Computer Science from Abdul Wali Khan University, Mardan, Pakistan. His master's thesis, titled "Route Optimization with Ant Colony Optimization (ACO)," has been published as a book in Germany and is available on Amazon. He also successfully completed the Huawei Technologies Pakistan Train the Trainer (TTT) Program. He has taught various subjects, including Computer Network Security, Artificial Intelligence, Machine Learning, Evolutionary Computing, and Cyber Security. He has authored or co-authored more than 50 research articles published in reputable journals, conferences, and book chapters. Notably, he recently introduced a novel routing protocol, E-ANTHOCNET, in the area of flying ad hoc networks. His research interests include Network System Security, Intrusion Detection, Intrusion Prevention, Cryptography, Optimization Techniques, WSN, IoT, Flying Ad Hoc Networks, and Machine Learning. He has served on the technical program committee for numerous international conferences, such as the *EAI International Conference on Future Intelligent Vehicular Technologies* in Islamabad, Pakistan, and the *2nd International Conference on Future Networks and Distributed Systems* in Amman, Jordan. He also contributed to the *International Workshop on Computational Intelligence and Cybersecurity in Emergent Networks (CICEN'21)*, held in conjunction with the *12th International Conference on Ambient Systems, Networks and Technologies (EUSPN2021)* in Leuven, Belgium, and was a committee member for the *International Workshop on Intelligent Systems for Sustainable Smart Cities* in New Delhi, India. In addition, he has served as the editor for around

20 books on various topics. He was the Special Session Chair at the *International Conference on Advances in Communication Technology and Computer Engineering (ICACTCE'22)* on the topic of "Fusion of Emerging Technologies: Communication Networks & Future Applications." He recently served as a Technical Program Committee Member at EAI MTYMEX 2024 in Vancouver, Canada, and is a Guest Editor for several international journals. He has held the position of General Chair for the *International Conference on Trends and Innovations in Smart Technologies (ICTIST'22)*, which was conducted virtually from London, United Kingdom. He is currently the General Chair for the *2nd International Conference on Trends and Innovations in Smart Technologies (ICTIST'24)*. Additionally, he was the President/General Chair for the *1st and 2nd International Conference on Emerging Trends & Innovation (ICETI)*. Notably, he has been invited as a technology expert on Pakistan National Television on several occasions.

Dr. Salma El Hajjami (Eng., Ph.D.) is an Assistant Professor and Researcher at the Faculty of Science, Ibn Zohr University, Agadir, Morocco, since 2021. She earned her Ph.D. in Computer Science in 2021 at the Laboratory of Artificial Intelligence, Data Science and Emerging Systems from ENSA, Sidi Mohammed Ben Abdellah University, Fez, Morocco. She is a Computer Science Engineer, who graduated in 2015 from the National School of Applied Sciences, Fez, Morocco. She has previous expertise acting in the Ministry of Interior Morocco as a Research and Development Engineer from 2017 to 2021. She is a member of the International Association of Engineers (IAENG) and the International Association of Online Engineering. She has made contributions in the fields of Social Big Data, Semantics Analytics, Anomaly Detection, and Imbalanced Big Data published at international conferences and journals. Her main research topics are Machine Learning, Deep Learning, Imbalanced Big Data, Data Science, and Blockchain. She has served and continues to serve on technical program and organizer committees of several conferences and also as a reviewer of numerous international journals.

Dr. Shashi Kant Gupta is a Post-Doctoral Fellow and a Researcher of Computer Science and Engineering at Eudoxia Research University, USA, in collaboration with Eudoxia Research Centre, India (ORCID: 0000-0001-6587-5607). He has completed his Ph.D. in CSE from Integral University, Lucknow, UP, India. He worked as an Assistant Professor in the Department of Computer Science and Engineering, PSIT, Kanpur, UP, India; worked as an Associate Professor at the School of Computer Applications, BBD University, Lucknow, UP, India; worked as an Assistant Professor in the Department of Computer Science and Engineering, Ambalika Institute of Management and Technology, Lucknow, UP, India; and also worked as a Senior Lecturer in the Department of IT, MCSCET, Lucknow, UP, India. He is currently working as the Founder and CEO of CREP PVT. LTD., Lucknow, UP, India. He has been a member of *IEEE Spectrum* and *IEEE Potentials Magazine* since 2019 and many more international organizations for research activities. He is an Editor-in-Chief of the *International Journal of Data Informatics and Intelligent Computing (IJDIIC)*. *IJDIIC* is an international open access, scholarly peer-reviewed journal publishing high-quality articles in all areas of data informatics and intelligent computing, especially current research, new concepts, innovative methods, and approaches for early detection and reporting new methods on basic and advanced aspects of data informatics and intelligent computing. He has published many research papers in reputed international journals with SCOPUS and SCI-indexed journals and published many papers in national and international conferences as well as in seminars. He has organized various faculty development programs, seminars, workshops, and short-term courses at the university level. His main research work focuses on performance enhancement through Cloud Computing, Big Data Analytics, IoT, and Computational Intelligence-based Education. He is currently working as a reviewer in various international journals like BJIT and many more. He is currently an editor in many CRC and Taylor and Francis Group publication books like *IoT Technologies, Big Data Solutions, Cloud Platforms, and Cybersecurity Techniques in Developing Smart Cities*; *AI-aided IoT Technologies and Applications in the Smart Business and Production*; *Designing Workforce Management Systems for Industry 4.0: Data-Centric and AI-Enabled Approaches*; *Smart Cities IoT Technologies, Big Data Solutions, Cloud Platforms, and Cybersecurity Techniques*; and *AI-Centric Modeling and Analytics Concepts, Technologies, and Applications.* He has published many Indian patents in the fields of information technology, computer science, and management. One Indian patent is under grant approval. He has many German patents with grants. He has more than 10 years of teaching experience, 2 years of Industrial Experience, and more than 2 years as CEO and Founder of a firm.

Hameedur Rahman received the BS and MS degrees in Software Engineering with Multimedia from the Limkokwing University of Creative Technology, Malaysia, and a Ph.D. degree in Computer Science from the Faculty of Information Science and Technology, University of Kebangsaan Malaysia, Bangi, Malaysia. He has 10 years of Industrial experience in multinational companies. He is currently an Associate Professor at AIR University, a Senior Research Member with the Center for Artificial Intelligence Technology, and Head of the Department of Computer Games Development. He received some international awards, including the Itex Bronze Medal of Innovation, Malaysia, and the Winner of NASA Space App and Virtual Reality Arena. His research interests include the areas of Augmented Reality, Virtual Reality, Image Processing, Cryptography, Natural Language Processing, Data Mining, Mobile Technology, Artificial Intelligence, Automation, and Medical Radiological Technology.

Dr. Thiagarajan Yogamoorthi (MIE, MISTE), Atal Mentor of Change, is currently working as an Associate Professor cum HOD in the Department of Electrical and Electronics Engineering, Christ College of Engineering and Technology, Puducherry, India. He has been teaching undergraduate students in Electrical and Electronics Engineering for the past 14 years. He is a member of the Board of Studies and also in the Doctoral Committee. Currently, he is serving as an Editorial Board Member and a Reviewer in various reputed journals, which include *Elsevier.* His research publication has been published in major indexed journals like ISI, Springer book proceedings, SCIE, and IEEE & ACEEE. He is a Fellow Member of the Solar Energy Society of India, a Member of the Institute of Engineers, a Senior Member of the IRD, a Life Member of ISTE, and a Member of various professional bodies. His research papers have reached the maximum reads of 5,000, via Research Gate. He has organized various faculty development programs, seminars, workshops, and short-term courses at the institution level in collaboration with various government bodies like Renewable Energy Agency, Puducherry, India; CIPAM; and NIPAM. His field of interest includes IoT in Renewable Energy, AI for E-Vehicles, Microbial Fuel Cell (PEM), Power Converters and Energy Conservation, Fuel Cell Technology, and Biomedical Engineering. He is the Recipient of the Best Faculty Award 2019, awarded by Vasavi International Trust. He has been selected as a Mentor for CSIR SRTP NEST 2020 (period: May–August 2020). To his credit, he has received one Indian Patent Grant, one Australian Innovation Patent Grant, and one Copyright Grant. He has presented papers in various national and international conferences. He has also participated in workshops, FDP, and other training programs. Currently, he has been selected as a mentor for ATAL Tinkerpreneur 2023, ranking in the 7th position continuously for two weeks out of 250 mentors.

Inam Ullah received a bachelor's degree in Electrical Engineering (Telecommunication) from the Department of Electrical Engineering, University of Science and Technology Bannu (USTB), KPK, Pakistan, in 2016 and master's and Ph.D. degrees in Information and Communication Engineering from the College of Internet of Things (IoT) Engineering, Hohai University (HHU), Changzhou Campus, 213022, China, in 2018 and 2022, respectively. He completed his postdoc with Brain Korea 2021 (BK21) at the Chungbuk Information Technology Education and Research Center, Chungbuk National University, Cheongju 28644, S Korea, from October 2022 to March 31, 2023. He is currently an Assistant Professor at the Department of Computer Engineering, Gachon University, S Korea. His research interests include Robotics, Internet of Things (IoT), Wireless Sensor Networks (WSNs), Underwater Communication and Localization, Underwater Sensor Networks (USNs), Artificial Intelligence (AI), Big Data, Deep Learning, etc. He has authored more than 70 peer-reviewed articles on various research topics. He is the reviewer of many prominent journals, including *IEEE Transactions on Industrial Informatics KSII Transactions on Internet & Information Systems*, *IEEE Transactions on Vehicular Technology*, *IEEE Transactions on Intelligent Transportation Systems*, *Transactions on Sustainable Computing*, *IEEE ACCESS*, *Sustainable Energy Technologies and Assessments*, *Future Generation Computer Systems (FGCS)*, *Computers and Electrical Engineering (Elsevier)*, *Internet of Things (IoT) Journal*, *Digital Communications & Networks (Elsevier)*, *Wireless Communication & Mobile Computing (WCMC)*, *Alexandria Engineering Journal Sensors*, *Electronics*, *Remote Sensing*, *Applied Sciences*, *Computational Intelligence and Neurosciences*, etc. His awards and honors include the Best Student Award from the University of Science and Technology Bannu (USTB), KPK, Pakistan, in 2015 and the Prime Minister Laptop Scheme Award from the University of Science and Technology Bannu (USTB), KPK, Pakistan, in April 2015. He has also received the Top-10 Students Award of the College of Internet of Things (IoT) Engineering, Hohai University, China, in June 2019; Top-100 Students Award of Hohai University (HHU), China, in June 2019; Jiangsu Province Distinguish International Students Award (30,000 RMB) in 2019–2020; Certificate of Recognition from Hohai University (HHU), China, in 2021 and 2022 both; Top-100 Students Award of Hohai University (HHU), China, in May 2022; Top-10 Outstanding Students Award, Hohai University (HHU), China, in June 2022; and Distinguished Alumni Award from University of Science and Technology Bannu (USTB), KPK, Pakistan, in October 2022.

Muhammad Adnan Khan (Senior Member, IEEE) is currently working as an Associate Professor in the School of Computing, Skyline University College, Sharjah, UAE. He earned his Ph.D. from ISRA University, Islamabad, Pakistan, by obtaining a scholarship award from the Higher Education Commission, Islamabad, Pakistan, in 2016. He also obtained his MS and BS degrees from the International Islamic University, Islamabad, Pakistan, by obtaining a scholarship award from the Punjab Information and Technology Board, Government of Punjab, Pakistan. Before joining Skyline University College, he has worked in various academic and industrial roles in Pakistan and Republic of Korea. He has been teaching graduate and undergraduate students in computer science and engineering for the past 15 years. Currently, he is guiding 5 Ph.D. scholars and 6 M.Phil. scholars. He has published more than 240 research articles with Cumulative JCR-IF 640+ in reputed international journals and international conferences. His research interests primarily include Machine Learning, Deep Learning, Applications of Computational Intelligence, Smart Health, Smart City, Federated Learning, Extreme Machine Learning, MUD, Image Processing and Medical Diagnosis, Channel Estimation in Multi-Carrier Communication Systems Using Soft Computing, etc.

Contributors

Srinithi A.
Kongu Engineering College
Perundurai, India

Aizhar Ali
Department of Computer Science
Shaheed Zulfikar Ali Bhutto Institute of Science and Technology
Islamabad, Pakistan

Nalini Kanta Barpanda
Department of Electronics
Sambalpur University
Burla, India

Santi Kumari Behera
Department of Computer Science and Engineering
VSSUT
Burla, India

Sharmila C.
SRM Institute of Science and Technology
Tiruchirappalli, India

Urvashi Dhanre
School of Mechanical Engineering
Vellore Institute of Technology
Vellore, India

Sajjad A. Ghauri
School of Engineering & Applied Sciences
ISRA University
Islamabad, Pakistan

Mohsen Ghorbian
Department of Computer Engineering, Qom Branch
Islamic Azad University
Qom, Iran

Saeid Ghorbian
Department of Molecular Genetics, Ahar Branch
Islamic Azad University
Ahar, Iran

Sadaf Hussain
Department of Computer Science
Lahore Garrison University
Lahore, Pakistan

Waqar Hussain
Department of Computer Science
Shaheed Zulfikar Ali Bhutto Institute of Science and Technology
Islamabad, Pakistan

Shahnaz Khademizadeh
Department of Knowledge & Information Science
Shahid Chamran University of Ahvaz
Ahvaz, Iran

Abdul Qadeer Khan
Department of Computer Engineering
National University of Technology
Islamabad, Pakistan

Ganesh Khekare
School of Computer Science and Engineering
Vellore Institute of Technology
Vellore, India

U.V. Kiran
Department of Human Development & Family Studies
School for Home Sciences
Babasaheb Bhimrao Ambedkar University
Lucknow, India

Dinesh Kumar B
Kongu Engineering College
Perundurai, India

Shahzad Latif
Department of Computer Science
Shaheed Zulfikar Ali Bhutto Institute of Science and Technology
Islamabad, Pakistan

Goutam Majumder
School of Computer Science and Engineering
Vellore Institute of Technology
Vellore, India

Mariyum Munir
Department of Computer Science
Shaheed Zulfikar Ali Bhutto Institute of Science and Technology
Islamabad, Pakistan

Nadiminti Venkata Ramana Murty
Department of Computer Science and Engineering (AI & ML)
Gayatri Vidya Parishad College for Degree and PG Courses (A)
Visakhapatnam, India

Abinaya N.
Hindustan Institute of Technology
Coimbatore, India

Jayadharshini P.
Kongu Engineering College
Perundurai, India

Ankita Patra
Department of Electronics
Sambalpur University
Burla, India

Santhiya S.
Kongu Engineering College
Perundurai, India

Ahthasham Sajid
Department of Cyber Security and Data Science
Riphah Institute of System Engineering
Riphah International University
Islamabad, Pakistan

Gopal Sakarkar
Department of Computer Science and Applications
Dr. Vishwanath Karad MIT World Peace University
Pune, India

Prabira Kumar Sethy
Department of Electronics and Communication Engineering
Guru Ghasidas Viswavidyalaya
Bilaspur, India

Shikha
Department of Human Development & Family Studies
School of Home Science
Babasaheb Bhimrao Ambedkar University
Lucknow, India

Fariha Shoukat
Department of Cyber Security and Data Science
Riphah Institute of System Engineering
Riphah International University
Islamabad, Pakistan

Tanweer Sohail
Department of Mathematics
University of Jhung
Jhung, Pakistan

Bhushan Vidhale
Department of Electronics and Telecommunication Engineering
G H Raisoni College of Engineering
Nagpur, India

Ganesh Yenurkar
Department of Computer Technology
Yeshwantrao Chavan College of Engineering
Nagpur, India

1 Sentiment Analysis of Users Tweets for Polarity Opinions Detection Using Deep Learning for Health Care Service

Shahnaz Khademizadeh, Ahthasham Sajid, Abdul Qadeer Khan, Fariha Shoukat, and Waqar Hussain

1.1 INTRODUCTION

Recent advances in information technology have led users to produce vast amounts of information, including online searches on social networks. Cultural and social networks have consistently encouraged and attracted thousands of users to subscribe—posting and sharing information about their ideas and opinions and participating in all-inclusive events online. Every day, we see a lot of posts, comments, and content uploaded by officials and users on these networks. Most of this information is stored in various text formats. On the other hand, applying techniques to discover and access information, habits, and behaviors of the audience of these networks in various cultural, social, political, marketing, etc., can be helpful. One of these techniques is data mining. Data mining is extracting useful information and patterns from large datasets. Moreover, latent information from a multitude of data, the process of which is growing exponentially. Remember the following text: Users of social networks like Facebook, LinkedIn, and Twitter have shared a large amount of personal information, which leads to storing large amounts of data on these networks. According to Tyagi and Tripathi (2019), social media platforms are widely used to connect and share information. Events from daily life are discussed on social media, and all users are free to comment on and discuss these events (Manguri et al., 2020). Also, information expressed through social media has influenced public sentiment (Depoux et al., 2020). Health Care Service is also one of the most biological virus outbreaks in the last two decades. For this reason, analyzing and gaining new insights from the data related to the Health Care Service on social media platforms can help health workers and government agencies take advantage of this data and understand people's reactions and emotions (Alsaeedi and Khan, 2019). Data mining facilities in social networks can be

DOI: 10.1201/9781003469896-1

used to discover the habits and behavior of social, cultural, political, etc., users. Data obtained from searching for keywords or phrases in social networks provides valuable information about the tastes, opinions, and thoughts of users on a particular topic or content (Injadat, Salo, and Nasif, 2016). Determining the interests and tastes of users based on social media data texts as well as examining the thematic importance of the content has recently become one of the most interesting and important research topics (Han and Lee, 2014) by other organizations, as well as officials, are interested in harnessing the pervasive capabilities and power of the vast amount of data available on social networks to make management decisions and policies ahead.

Since social media analytics are very popular among users and have become an important topic for knowledge discovery, Sentiment analysis helps to understand human emotions because it can explore people's behaviors when users spend on these social media applications (Ji et al., 2016). Extracting human emotion and entertainment from large-scale social media networks is essential for international public influence, business decisions, and policy development (Chung et al., 2015). Therefore, sentiment analysis is a powerful tool for understanding the most important events and trends (Alamoodi et al., 2021). The present study intends to first analyze the feelings of Twitter users about Health Care Service by clustering their feelings.

The rapid growth of the use of the Internet and social networks has caused the creation of a large number of texts containing people's opinions that could not be recorded in the past. Opinions and opinions contain valuable information that by analyzing them, one can understand the tendencies and preferences of people and identify positive and negative opinions on various issues. Knowing people's opinions is very important for many matters related to decision-making. The analysis of users' opinions and feelings about the news and measures taken in the field of Health Care Service can be used for policy making and national macro-decisions. Due to the importance of analyzing users' opinions and, generally, the content created by them, in recent years, the field of sentiment analysis has attracted the attention of researchers. In the past, traditional methods such as questionnaires have been used to collect people's opinions and feelings on various issues, but today, by using the tools that social networks provide to their users, people can easily expose their opinions to others. The research was conducted with the aim of investigating the positive, negative, and neutral opinions of Twitter social network users using tweets published about Health Care Service. Previous studies have presented different approaches to analyze user sentiment in social media data (Singh et al., 2020, 2022; Wang et al., 2018; Pham and Le, 2018; Aflakparast et al., 2018; Schmidt and Wiegand, 2017). Therefore, the present study was conducted with the aim of investigating the positive, negative, and neutral opinions of Twitter social network users using tweets published about Health Care Service. To achieve this goal, the sentiment analysis technique was used in the fields of deep learning and machine learning.

1.1.1 Related Works

Data mining and social networks have been used rapidly today; hence, it has become desirable for researchers, policymakers, and marketers to discover hidden knowledge to make decisions and plans. Especially recently, many studies have been conducted inside and outside the country in the field of data mining applications in virtual and social networks, an example of which is mentioned below:

In a review activity, Ismaili and Zahid (2014) briefly introduced the methods and challenges of text mining in social networks.

Pikri, Yacoubi, and Taheri (2014), as one of the few research studies in the Persian language in the field of text mining, using text mining technique and content analysis, studied the phenomenon of Morteza Pasha'i's death in the Twitter social network and the published tweets in this connection included 17,714 tweets in five classification categories and analyzed the correlation between the categories with the characteristics of the users.

Sohrabi et al. (2015), in research that aimed to provide a model for analyzing the behavior of social network users using data-mining methods, addressed a case of a social network in Iran, which resulted in a better understanding of user behavior patterns. It ended up in social networks.

Tawakli and Rafe (2015) presented a method to analyze the comments below the news on news sites according to the news text. In this regard, by using grammatical features of texts such as nouns and verbs, as well as analyzing the emotional load of the sentence, it has been tried to discover the relationship between the opinion and the news and the writer's point of view regarding the subject of the news text.

Abbasi et al. (2016), in research to provide a model for categorizing the feelings of book buyers from the Amazon site, which was carried out using a combined approach, concluded that the recommendation system can automatically identify positive and negative comments. Classify with more than 80% accuracy.

Badr, Mohammad Ismail, and Heydari in research aimed at classifying the target users of the central library.

The Isfahan University of Technology has identified their behaviors and information needs by using a neural network technique and a questionnaire. The least effective component is gaining a scientific point of view and competing with equal people. Most of the information sources needed by library users are translation of Latin books, and their least need are research reports and plans. The most critical obstacle to their information is not having access to the proper internet and the least influential factor is the troublesome use of resources. The most information-seeking skill of users is their awareness of their information needs and the access channels to it, and the least influential component is the ability to recognize the importance of the information obtained from searches and its correspondence with their information needs. The ability of librarians and information specialists to retrieve information and their knowledge of information resources and services are the most influential factors in meeting information needs; on the other hand, familiarity with a variety of information resources and service types in their field of expertise and the ability to use digital files instead of physical library resources are the least effective factors. Based on their requirements and information-seeking activities, target library users can be categorized using the neural network technique in data mining, according to the goal and conclusions of the current study.

In research aiming to focus on the study category, the Serbian Cultural and Information Institute website was subjected to detailed text mining using thematic clustering. After the topic clustering and text mining method, while identifying prominent and less essential topic clusters, the importance of this topic among Tebian network users was investigated. Considering the cultural nature of the explanation and the matter of reading and studying, searching for related key phrases will provide the most results in the subject category of culture with 26% and 18%, respectively. Considering the virtual and electronic nature of the Tebian site, the electronic education section of this site must cover this deficiency by producing more educational content. Despite the high number of results obtained in the subject class of the society, the results in the whole network for the category of reading books are very few, and this shows the need for more activity in Tabayan to improve this neglected culture in the country.

1.1.2 Related Work

Pourgholam Ali, Kahani, and Asgarian (2019) in a study they conducted with the aim of using big data technology for opinion mining, the results obtained indicate that the proposed framework for opinion mining worked efficiently and not only for high volumes but also in Volumes of about 20 MB we see a 100-fold increase in efficiency. This coefficient increases more noticeably in higher volumes.

Mohammadi, Yazdian Dehkordi, and Nemat Bakhsh (2019) in research that was conducted with the aim of identifying implicit features using the syntactic rules of the Persian language and attribute clustering. The evaluations performed on the real data and extracted from the users' comments on the Digi-Kala site show that the method presented in this article has achieved a better reading rate and accuracy than the previous works.

Lazard et al. (2015) in a study supported by the Center for Disease Control and Prevention of the United States of America, using the method of text exploration and analysis, investigated the spread of public panic through text mining of live tweets among users and came to the conclusion that public opinion is highly concerned about the symptoms and duration of the Ebola virus, how the virus is transmitted, and how to protect the body while traveling.

Banus et al. in a study investigated how to improve strategies for generating secondary information such as effective clustering and classification algorithms based on probabilistic models and using text mining techniques to discover implicit knowledge in texts. They used social networks. This study has focused mainly on text mining methodology with emphasis on the number of clusters used, execution time, and accuracy of text mining activity.

Kim and Sin (2016) in a study examined different social network systems used by undergraduate students and librarians of university libraries to obtain information and how to evaluate the information obtained from these networks in a scientific environment by comparing habits and methods. The two collections were discussed together so that they could measure the distance created between them. The selected sample of students was 1,355 people and the selected sample of librarians was 189 people, and the result is that the social network system used and the purpose of using this network were similar for both groups, but there was a big gap in terms of the strategies used to obtain information.

Al-Daihani and Abrahams (2016) investigated the tweet database of 10 university libraries, including 23,707 tweets, 17,848 bookmarks, and 5,974 retweets using the text mining method and stated that with this method, it is possible to make appropriate strategic planning and make appropriate management decisions. Used to provide ideal services for clients.

Blue Ergaz et al. investigated and monitored the discussions of Twitter social network forums using the text mining method in relation to the effects of the discussions on the decisions made by public health organizations.

After putting up a user modeling framework that groups texts in social media into pertinent categories. Kang and Lee (2017) conducted research to model user interest in mass communication websites using news media and Wikipedia. They came to the conclusion that by employing Wikipedia as a foreign knowledge base in their modeling, the semantic gap between social media and news media is lowered in the news media. The suggested approach, which makes use of Wikipedia properties, outperforms other current techniques for determining users' interests from social media.

In their research, Carvalho and Plastino (2021) concluded that sentiment analysis of informal short texts, such as tweets, is a challenging task due to their specific characteristics. Much effort has been made in the Twitter sentiment analysis literature to achieve an effective and efficient representation of tweets. In this context, different types of features have been proposed and used, from simple n-gram display to the above features to word embedding. Therefore, using the relevant set of 22 sets of tweets, they present a complete evaluation of the features using different supervised learning algorithms. Not only a rich set of meta-features that have been investigated in advanced studies but also a significant set of pre-trained word embedding models have been evaluated. Also, we evaluated and analyzed the effect of combining these distinct types of features to identify which combination might provide the main information in the task of polarity detection in Twitter sentiment analysis. For this purpose, they used different strategies for combination, such as feature combination and group learning techniques, and showed that tweet sentiment recognition benefits from the combination of different types of features presented in the literature.

Barreto et al. (2021) use a comprehensive set of 22 datasets from various areas and five classification methods to assess the performance of current language models in identifying emotions expressed in tweets. Static and contextual representations are included in the evaluation. Transformer-based auto-encoder models provide the contexts, and these models are also configurable with a variety of techniques according to the language mask model task.

1.1.3 Summary of Backgrounds

In the past years, the importance and role of data mining in social networks has increased rapidly. The research findings in this field show that among the techniques of sentiment analysis in network data mining social media is used to get users' attitudes. Therefore, in Table 1.1, a summary of the studies related to this research is given.

TABLE 1.1
Summary of Related Works

Research Findings	Data Collection and Analysis Method	Statistical and Sample Population	Issue	Researcher (year)
User clustering into four clusters: indifferent, weak, ordinary, and bigoted fans	K average	100 social network users	Evaluate people's entertainment on social networks	Khobzi and Teimourpour (2015)
Algorithms with models three-classes and five-classes have been used	New Bay is the closest neighbor to the decision-making association rules	20,000 users of a social network	Predict people's personalities by exploring social interactions on Facebook	Ortigosa et al. (2014)
Identify four clusters of users	Decrease in MCA mean K	Facebook users	User clustering	van Dam and van de Velden (2014)
Provide a personalized search system	Algorithms GEW 3C	–	Dynamic profiles for website personalization	Hawalah and Fasli (2015)
Presenting theoretical and practical concepts	Statistical methods questionnaire	320 members of different social networks	Loyalty to the social network	Tsiotsou (2015)
This study provides a multivariate emotional behavior analysis of social network users that allows users to cluster	PCA - similarity Distance - similarity	49 users of a 556 Chinese social network	Clustering social network users based on emotional behavior	Jiang et al. (2014)
Provide a model for identifying groups on the social network	Decision tree or graph	–	New method clustering in social networks	Zhao and Zhang (2011)

By examining the existing backgrounds in social networks, there was no research that analyzed sentiment in the Twitter social network in the context of Health Care Service.

1.2 METHODOLOGY

1.2.1 Conceptual Model of Research

The steps of the current research are briefly given below.

Step 1: Choose the social network that publishes the most information about Health Care Service.
Instagram Twitter or..
Step 2: Data extraction from social networks is done in two ways:
Via api via bot or kroll
Step 3: Data cleaning and data normalization
Step 4: Examining positive and negative sentences
Step 5: Implementation of the appropriate algorithm

The steps of conducting sentiment analysis research in social networks

Step 1: Choosing the social network that publishes the most information about Health Care Service.

Step 2: Data extraction: Data extraction from social networks is done in two ways:

a. Use through api (the site itself provides this possibility in a limited way) and/or
b. It is used through a robot or crawling data (a robot or crawler is written to receive information from social networks). The limitation of this method is that it does not provide us with the location or part of the content.

Step 3: Data cleaning and data normalization: According to the existing data, they are normalized or cleaned, additional information is removed, a number is assigned to it, and the data is used for the next step. Getting ready

Step 4: According to the existing dataset, the existing data is split, prepositions are removed, and positive or negative sentences are checked inside the text.

Step 5: According to the cleaned data, the available algorithms are implemented on these data and the appropriate algorithm is used in the article.

1.2.1.1 Data Collection and Pre-Processing

Collecting data for research is not an easy task, although it may seem simple at first. But there are hypotheses and decisions that we have to consider. There are two general types of data: training data (to train the classification model) and test data (to test the classification). But before discussing them, we will discuss Twitter's programming interfaces.

1.2.1.2 Twitter Interfaces

Twitter has two user interfaces: the two-API Rest API and the two-API Streaming API. Long-term connections are supported via streaming API, which can deliver data promptly. Although the Rest API can only download a set amount of data each day and only enables short-term connections, there is a threshold restriction for this download (see Rest Regardless of the time, the API provides access to Twitter data, including status updates and user profiles; however, data is only retained for a maximum of seven days.

Therefore, Rest's access is limited to the data before one week. It also provides access to data in an accumulated form, while the Streaming API provides access to data from the time the tweet was sent.

To create a suitable model, we need a relatively adequate amount of training data. To train the classification model, we used the Twitter dataset. This dataset includes tweets that are categorized into three categories: positive, negative, and neutral. This dataset contains 1,600,000 tweets collected by Twitter APIs; despite the fact that the dataset refers to the neutral class, our goal is to create a binary category, so only we consider tweets that have positive and negative polarities.

1.2.2 Data Preprocessing

Before creating the category model on the data, a series of pre-processing should be done on the data because much of the information in this dataset has practically no conceptual load and does not have an effect on the overall accuracy of the category, which in the steps we will discuss below.

1.2.3 Data Cleaning

In this process, unnecessary information or information that has been collected incorrectly is deleted, which includes:

- **Converting the HTML format to the general text format**: with the checks done on the data, some HTML tags have appeared in the text format, which should be converted to its general format.
- **Removal of reference or @mention**: Although @mentions mention useful information for users, they have no effect on the category. Therefore, in the second step, we delete all the @mention signs in the dataset.

  URL source links: The third part of the cleaning process is dealing with source links. These links also convey useful information, but for sentiment analysis, these links can be ignored.
- **Hashtags and numbers**: Sometimes the text used with the hashtag can provide useful information about the tweet. Removing all existing hashtags may cause the loss of some useful information, so we decided to keep the text unchanged and only remove the # hashtag sign.

Preprocessing and cleaning are important in terms of computational time and classifier accuracy because additional data may slow down the learning process, the classifier may learn irrelevant information, and the efficiency of the system will decrease completely. The overview of the dataset before and after removing irrelevant information is shown in Figures 1.1 and 1.2.

1.2.3.1 Basic Parameters

Bengio defines basic parameters as follows: we choose a basic parameter as a value for algorithm A before applying it to actual data. However, the learning algorithm itself does not directly choose the feature in the chosen algorithm. It means choosing the most appropriate value and algorithm among algorithms and values. Basic parameters can be continuous, such as the learning rate, or discrete, such as the number of neurons in each neural network layer. We consider an example to show

	A	B	C	D	E	F	G
1	0	1.47E+09	Mon Apr (	NO_QUER	_TheSpeci	@switchfoot http://twitpic.com/2y1zl - Awww, that's a bummer. You shoulda got David Carr of Third Day to do it. ;D	
2	0	1.47E+09	Mon Apr (	NO_QUER	scotthami	is upset that he can't update his Facebook by texting it... and might cry as a result School today also. Blah!	
3	0	1.47E+09	Mon Apr (	NO_QUER	mattycus	@Kenichan I dived many times for the ball. Managed to save 50% The rest go out of bounds	
4	0	1.47E+09	Mon Apr (	NO_QUER	ElleCTF	my whole body feels itchy and like its on fire	
5	0	1.47E+09	Mon Apr (	NO_QUER	Karoli	@nationwideclass no, it's not behaving at all. i'm mad. why am i here? because I can't see you all over there.	
6	0	1.47E+09	Mon Apr (	NO_QUER	joy_wolf	@Kwesidei not the whole crew	
7	0	1.47E+09	Mon Apr (	NO_QUER	mybirch	Need a hug	
8	0	1.47E+09	Mon Apr (	NO_QUER	coZZ	@LOLTrish hey long time no see! Yes.. Rains a bit ,only a bit LOL , I'm fine thanks , how's you ?	
9	0	1.47E+09	Mon Apr (	NO_QUER	2Hood4Hc	@Tatiana_K nope they didn't have it	
10	0	1.47E+09	Mon Apr (	NO_QUER	mimismo	@twittera que me muera ?	
11	0	1.47E+09	Mon Apr (	NO_QUER	erinx3lear	spring break in plain city... it's snowing	
12	0	1.47E+09	Mon Apr (	NO_QUER	pardonlau	I just re-pierced my ears	
13	0	1.47E+09	Mon Apr (	NO_QUER	TLeC	@caregiving I couldn't bear to watch it. And I thought the UA loss was embarrassing	
14	0	1.47E+09	Mon Apr (	NO_QUER	robrobbie	@octolinz16 It it counts, idk why I did either. you never talk to me anymore	
15	0	1.47E+09	Mon Apr (	NO_QUER	bayofwolv	@smarrison i would've been the first, but i didn't have a gun. not really though, zac snyder's just a doucheclown.	
16	0	1.47E+09	Mon Apr (	NO_QUER	HairByJes	@iamjazzyfizzle I wish I got to watch it with you!! I miss you and @iamlilnicki how was the premiere?!	
17	0	1.47E+09	Mon Apr (	NO_QUER	lovesongv	Hollis' death scene will hurt me severely to watch on film wry is directors cut not out now?	
18	0	1.47E+09	Mon Apr (	NO_QUER	armotley	about to file taxes	
19	0	1.47E+09	Mon Apr (	NO_QUER	starkissed	@LettyA ahh ive always wanted to see rent love the soundtrack!!	
20	0	1.47E+09	Mon Apr (	NO_QUER	gi_gi_bee	@FakerPattyPattz Oh dear. Were you drinking out of the forgotten table drinks?	

FIGURE 1.1 Overview of the dataset before removing irrelevant information.

	A	B	C	D	E	F	G
1	0	1.47E+09	Mon Apr (	NO_QUER	_TheSpeci	www, that's a bummer. You shoulda got David Carr of Third Day to do it. ;D	
2	0	1.47E+09	Mon Apr (	NO_QUER	scotthami	is upset that he can't update his Facebook by texting it... and might cry as a result School today also. Blah!	
3	0	1.47E+09	Mon Apr (	NO_QUER	mattycus	I dived many times for the ball. Managed to save 50% The rest go out of bounds	
4	0	1.47E+09	Mon Apr (	NO_QUER	ElleCTF	my whole body feels itchy and like its on fire	
5	0	1.47E+09	Mon Apr (	NO_QUER	Karoli	no, it's not behaving at all. i'm mad. why am i here? because I can't see you all over there.	
6	0	1.47E+09	Mon Apr (	NO_QUER	joy_wolf	not the whole crew	
7	0	1.47E+09	Mon Apr (	NO_QUER	mybirch	Need a hug	
8	0	1.47E+09	Mon Apr (	NO_QUER	coZZ	hey long time no see! Yes.. Rains a bit ,only a bit LOL , I'm fine thanks , how's you ?	
9	0	1.47E+09	Mon Apr (	NO_QUER	2Hood4Hc	nope they didn't have it	
10	0	1.47E+09	Mon Apr (	NO_QUER	mimismo	que me muera ?	
11	0	1.47E+09	Mon Apr (	NO_QUER	erinx3lear	spring break in plain city... it's snowing	
12	0	1.47E+09	Mon Apr (	NO_QUER	pardonlau	I just re-pierced my ears	
13	0	1.47E+09	Mon Apr (	NO_QUER	TLeC	I couldn't bear to watch it. And I thought the UA loss was embarrassing	
14	0	1.47E+09	Mon Apr (	NO_QUER	robrobbie	It it counts, idk why I did either. you never talk to me anymore	
15	0	1.47E+09	Mon Apr (	NO_QUER	bayofwolv	i would've been the first, but i didn't have a gun. not really though, zac snyder's just a doucheclown.	
16	0	1.47E+09	Mon Apr (	NO_QUER	HairByJes	I wish I got to watch it with you!! I miss you and @iamlilnicki how was the premiere?!	
17	0	1.47E+09	Mon Apr (	NO_QUER	lovesongv	Hollis' death scene will hurt me severely to watch on film wry is directors cut not out now?	
18	0	1.47E+09	Mon Apr (	NO_QUER	armotley	about to file taxes	
19	0	1.47E+09	Mon Apr (	NO_QUER	starkissed	ahh ive always wanted to see rent love the soundtrack!!	
20	0	1.47E+09	Mon Apr (	NO_QUER	gi_gi_bee	Oh dear. Were you drinking out of the forgotten table drinks?	

FIGURE 1.2 Overview of the dataset after removing irrelevant information.

the difference between the primary and other parameters. We want to teach a polynomial function for a specific function; the polynomial function is as follows, where M is the polynomial degree, and W_i is the polynomial coefficients $w = w_1, w_2, w_3, \ldots w_n$, M must be set manually and determined before training the polynomial function. As a result, M is a fundamental parameter. On the other hand, W_i, which are polynomial coefficients, depends on the training phase. In some cases, such as neural networks, the number of fundamental parameters can be relatively high (dozens or more), complicating the problem.

1.2.3.2 Model Selection

Different learning models show the number of free parameters and complexities that need adjustment (Lee et al., 2017). Along with the model itself, the parameters of the model must be adjusted. The general goal in this field is to choose the values of the free parameters to have the best prediction performance on new data (Nair and Hinton, 2020).

The training set is not a good indicator for evaluating the predicted performance from different parameter values. Instead, if there is enough dataset, the dataset can be divided into three parts. The model is trained with the first part, and the values of the basic parameters called the training set (Nair and Hinton, 2020). The second part is not used for training, but it is used to adjust the values of the basic parameters of the model so that the values can be compared to different basic parameters and choose one of the best ones for prediction. This independent dataset is called a validation dataset. Finally, a third part of the test data is needed to evaluate the model in terms of generalization. This means that the dataset used with validation to select the final model is no longer entirely independent of the model, and overfitting may occur on the validation data (Nair and Hinton, 2020).

Cross-validation is another technique separating the data into two sets for training and testing. This technique is also applied when a small dataset is needed for training, yet a significant amount of data is needed. Although various validation techniques exist, they all work on the same principle. One popular kind is called "k-fold validation," where the dataset is split into k sections, of which $k-1$ is used to train the model, and the remaining group is used to evaluate the model. This process is repeated for each category in such a way that, in the end, all the categories have been used once to evaluate the model (Nair and Hinton, 2020). The average performance of all the performances is the model's performance. In addition to the validation error, a method for calculating the general error, computational aspects may also be used for the basic parameters. There are various methods for optimizing the basic parameters. Like coordinate search, search with multiple resolutions, network search, or random search, the main weakness of these techniques is that the number of configurations increases exponentially with the increase in the number of basic parameters. For example, for six basic parameters, each of which can take five different values, this value is equal to 320,000 different combinations that can be considered for it.

On the other hand, network search can be implemented in parallel, and the advantage of this method is the ability to run different combinations on different computers. Random search is a suitable alternative, in which all parameters change simultaneously compared to grid search, and each parameter is independently sampled from a prior distribution (for example, a uniform distribution within the target space). Random sampling can be more efficient than network search; however, the qualitative analysis of the results is more complicated.

1.2.3.3 Examination of Over-Fitting and Under-Fitting

As mentioned, machine algorithms aim to maximize prediction accuracy on new data. This accuracy is not considered for training data. If the model is entirely suitable for the training data, the prediction accuracy for new data could be better. For a better understanding, we will give an example. Let us map the order of M. The value of M must be determined to determine the complexity of this linear model. Figure 1.1 shows several orders of high degree $M=9$, which suits the training data. However, it fluctuates wildly and exhibits very realistic performance, making it perform poorly on test data, called the over-fitting problem (Grishik et al., 2019). Other lower-degree polynomials $M=0$, $M=1$ are not complex enough, so the error increases on both the training and test data. This is called the under-fitting problem.

The implementation of these algorithms has been using the Cross library. We used different configurations for convolutional networks. In the training and evaluation phase, we used 90% of the data in the training set as training data for training the model and 10% as the evaluation set to adjust the model parameters. Then, we made different categories on them. Below are the results of applying these categories to the training and validation data.

1.2.4 Convolutional Neural Networks

The results obtained in the Results section are for convolution networks with different filter sizes and binary classification, and we will first configure each of them.

1.2.5 Social Network

The use of social networks and taking advantage of their extensive interactive features has become widespread today. It has attracted the attention of many audiences, so the users of social networks spend most of their time-saving. Their knowledge is produced and disseminated (Pourgholam et al., 2019). The term "social network" is not widely used, nor is its definition set in stone. Boyd and Ellison provided the following definition of social networks: "Social networking sites are web-based services that enable users to share a list of other users, see a list of people who are related to them and those whom they were introduced to through other users in the system, and spend time with them (Boyd and EIlison, 2007). Social networks around the world. They have become essential sources of information and an environment to follow and spread tendencies, news, and ideas (Kang and Lee, 2017). Therefore, social networks are defined as a set of relationships that people with interest Mendi connects the same.

Social network analysis can provide helpful insight by showing simple patterns of relationships based on a single event from data obtained through questionnaires, document analysis, sentiment analysis, etc. It will tell us about the network structure and each node's role in the shortest time and with the lowest cost.

1.2.6 Data Mining

As mentioned earlier, the opinions and opinions of others can be very vital when making a decision and choosing an option from several options. Viewpoints are the center of human activities (Liu, 2012). Virtual social networks represent a new generation of social interactions that has been able to make a good place in people's lives. Considering the ever-increasing scope of influence and influence of these networks, the problem of recognizing the behavioral patterns of their users has become one of the interesting research topics. Content sharing helps people to share useful information. Receiving public opinions about social events, marketing activities, and product priorities has attracted the attention of scientific communities and the business world (Cambria and Hussain, 2015). Nowadays, if someone wants to buy a product, there are numerous options available, it is no longer limited to the opinions of family and friends because users' opinions and discussions about various products are available on the web. For an organization, there is no need to conduct surveys and focus groups because such information is abundantly available on the Internet. However, finding and evaluating opinions is a challenging task due to the range and variety of opinions. Every site usually has a large number of textual comments that are not easy to decipher. In general, extracting and summarizing such information is not an easy task, so automatic sentiment analysis systems are needed (Liu, 2012). Social networks such as Twitter, Amazon, and TripAdvisor have increased the power of social networks to express opinions about services, products, and events. Today, individuals and organizations increasingly use the content of these media to make decisions (Liu, 2015).

Despite the increasing growth of this volume of textual information, it is necessary to have tools for organizing, retrieving, and extracting useful knowledge from this data. In this regard, extensive research has been done on data mining methods. The main reason for using data mining methods for textual documents is to structure them (Keshavarzian and Barardekht, 2016). The available methods for structuring texts are classification methods and clustering methods. The combination of text mining methods with structuring methods provides powerful tools for exploring useful patterns in text collections. Text-mining and big data analysis are the result of a knowledge discovery process through large databases such as social networks, whose purpose is to recognize unknown patterns and generate knowledge. The face is defined as:

Information retrieval: The process of finding documents containing answers to research questions and the process of finding the answers themselves is not included. In order to reach this objective, statistical methods are utilized to automatically process textual data and compare it with the presented questions.

Natural language processing: It means the possibility of using written materials in natural languages (such as English and Farsi) and understanding these writings by the machine. These techniques can be used in summarizing, text mining, and querying Persian languages.

Information extraction: The purpose of this is to obtain specific information from text documents, which are stored in patterns similar to databases to be used in the future.

Data mining helps organizations to discover and predict patterns, trends, and future behaviors by exploring the data of a system and make better decisions. Data mining provides an automatic and predictive analysis using the analysis of past events and answers questions that were not possible to answer in the past or required a lot of time. Data mining tools discover and predict hidden patterns that experts may not consider and find because these information and patterns are beyond their expectations. The extracted patterns can be a relationship between the characteristics and specifications of the system such as the type of demand and the type of customer, future predictions based on the characteristics of the system, rules (if-then) between system variables, classification and clustering of similar objects and records in one system and another (Chen, Han and Yu, 1996).

Preprocessing is the most time-consuming stage of the knowledge discovery process, but due to the direct effect of data preparation on the quality of data mining results, this stage is necessary. The data available in the real world may not have the necessary quality to start data mining, for example, the existence of "noise", "duplicate data in the data", "missing values", and "outliers". "Noise" makes it necessary to perform the pre-processing step. Also, due to data collection from different databases, these data may have different formats. Performing data mining on the data that is of low quality will lead to low-quality results. Therefore, it can be said that performing the pre-processing stage on the data before data mining will improve the performance of the whole process. Therefore, it is necessary to choose methods suitable for pre-processing should be given special attention.

1.2.7 Sentiment Analysis

Today, a large amount of textual data is available for processing, and the amount of these data increases every year (Niknam and NikNafs, 2015). Textual data is one of the most important forms of unstructured data. This type of data is a large reservoir of information from which we can extract appropriate content. One way to extract information from textual data is sentiment analysis.

Sentiment analysis is one of the branches of data mining science. Therefore, first, the purpose of data mining is examined, which includes exploratory data analysis, discovery of patterns, rules and algorithms, predictive modeling, and search for deviations.

As previously said, the study of sentiment analysis examines people's beliefs, emotions, assessments, and attitudes about various entities, including goods, services, companies, individuals, problems, occasions, subjects, and their attributes. It evaluates (Liu, 2012).

1.2.8 Machine Learning Approaches

Machine learning approaches can be generally divided into two parts: (1) Supervised machine learning approaches. (2) Unsupervised machine learning approaches. The supervised machine learning approach is a type of learning in which the input and output are known, and there is a supervisor who provides information to the learner, and thus the system tries to perform a function from the unsupervised machine learning approach. Input to output is covered. In unsupervised machine learning approach, unlike supervised learning, there is no specific data in advance, and the goal is not the input and output communication, but only their classification is important, and it is the learner who should be in the data to look for a specific structure (Liu, 2015).

1.2.9 Dictionary Approach

A dictionary-based approach is a basic approach for text analysis. This approach uses a dictionary or text where each word in the text is related to a specific idea. By using the words in the text, a weighted average of the emotion scores of the text is presented (Wong, 2017).

In the dictionary or dictionaries, the set of words are labeled and scored based on the feelings hidden in them; that is, the words with positive feelings are shown with positive numbers, and the words with negative feelings are shown with negative numbers. Due to the importance of dictionaries in sentiment analysis and opinion analysis, some dictionaries are introduced.

1.2.9.1 Opinion Search Dictionary

It is a polarity-based vocabulary resource that was introduced by Wilson et al. (2005). This developed dictionary is a collection of multi-dimensional question-and-answer data that includes mental expressions and sentences. In this dictionary, each sentence is labeled based on positive, negative, and neutral tendency classes.

1.2.9.2 Dictionary of Bing Liu's Thought

This dictionary was introduced by Liu (2012) and he also used it in several other researches. This dictionary is also based on polarity and consists of 2006 positive words and 4,683 negative words. This dictionary also includes misspelled words and slang words.

1.2.9.3 AFINN Dictionary

This dictionary was created by Nielsen (2011) and its focus is on the languages used in the context of blogs. The list of words in this dictionary includes vulgar and obscene words as well as surnames and terms specific to the web. This dictionary contains 2,477 English words, and the scores of positive words are between 1 and 5, and the scores of negative words are between −1 and −5. Therefore, it is suitable for estimating the strength of an opinion.

- Wordnet, Wordnet Effect, and Traditional Wordnet are dictionaries that can also be used for sentiment analysis.

1.2.10 Combined Approach

In some research, a combination method has been used. In this way, the data that are initially determined based on the method based on the dictionary of their emotional load, are used as input data for training the model in the machine learning algorithms in the supervised method. (Filho and Pardo, 2013).

1.2.11 Steps of Feeling Analysis or Opinion Analysis

The process of sentiment analysis in order to discover knowledge is carried out in different stages, which include the following in order.

Target identification, data selection, data preparation, including data cleaning, adopting the best data-mining method, implementing data-mining, i.e. applying the algorithm, evaluating and validating the findings, using the results, and confirming Discovered knowledge and decision-making based on discovered knowledge.

1.2.12 Common Categories in Sentiment Analysis

Various techniques have been presented to analyze emotions, which are shown in Figure 1.3. A summary of these methods.

In the following, we introduce a number of common categories in sentiment analysis.

1.2.12.1 Possible Categories

Three possible categories are as follows:

1.2.12.1.1 Simple Biz Classification

This type of classification is the simplest and most widely used type of classification. In this type of classification, the probability of the class is recognized based on the distribution of words in the text.

Relationship 1:

$$p(\text{label} \mid \text{features}) = p(\text{label}) \times p(\text{features} \mid \text{label}) / p(\text{features})$$

p (label): the initial probability of that label or the probability that a random feature belongs to that label.

p (features|label): the probability of a feature provided that it belongs to the label.

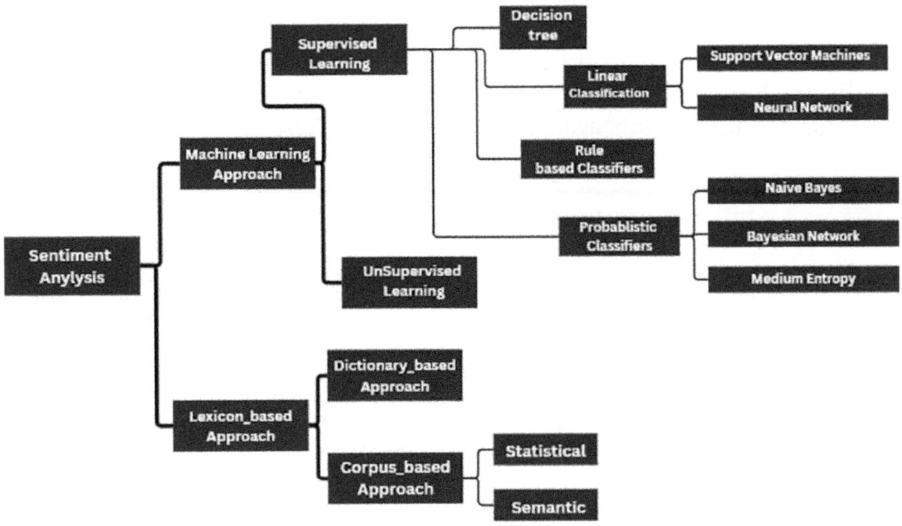

FIGURE 1.3 Sentiment analysis techniques (Pandey et al., 2017).

p (features): the initial probability of that feature.

If the features are independent of each other, the above formula can be written as follows:

Relationship 2:

$$p(\text{label} \mid \text{features}) = p(\text{label}) \times p(f1 \mid \text{label}) \ \ldots \ \times p(fn \mid \text{label})/p(\text{features})$$

1.2.12.2 Neural Networks

Neural networks are new computing systems and methods for machine learning, displaying knowledge and finally applying the obtained knowledge to predict the output responses of complex systems. The main idea of such networks is inspired by how the neurobiological system works to process data and information for learning and creating knowledge. The key aspect of this concept is to develop new structures for the information processing system. This system is comprised of numerous interconnected processing elements known as neurons, which collaborate to solve problems and transmit information via synapses (electromagnetic communication). In this network, if one cell is damaged, the rest of the cells can compensate for its absence and contribute to its reconstruction. These networks are capable of learning. For example, the cells remember by applying irritation to the touch nerve cells. They get that they do not go towards the hot object, and with this algorithm, the system learns to correct its error. Learning in these systems is done adaptively, that is, by using examples, the weight of synapses. It changes in such a way that the system produces the correct response when new inputs are given. In Figures 1.4 and 1.5, you can observe the workings of neural networks and their resemblance to the functioning of the biological nervous system. The neural network is represented by the vector x, which in sentiment analysis problems is the number of repetitions of the i-th word in the document. W is the series of weights assigned to neurons, which are from these Inputs that are used to calculate a function.

Multi-layer neural networks are used in more complex problems that require non-linear classification. The learning process is more complicated because the errors must recursively propagate through different layers.

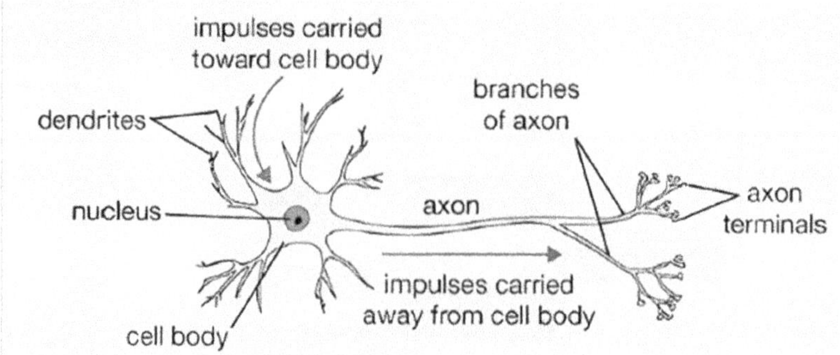

FIGURE 1.4 Human neural network and how it works (Yu et al., 2008).

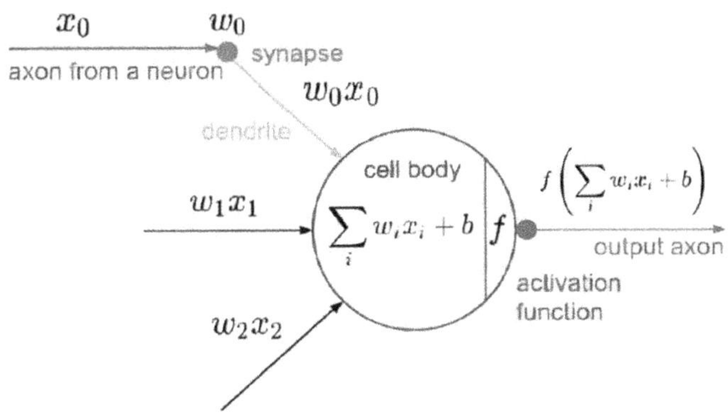

FIGURE 1.5 The functioning of neural networks and their similarity with the human network.

Neural networks for document classification produce good results for complex domains and are suitable for any type of data, whether continuous or discrete. The test stage of neural networks is high-speed, unlike its training stage. Also, neural networks can be implemented in parallel because each element can calculate its input value from the stored value independently of the other. This parallel implementation will increase the speed of calculations. One of the disadvantages of neural networks is the high cost of calculations, which uses a lot of processor and memory; another disadvantage is the possibility of overlearning. Understanding how neural networks work is difficult for an average number of users (Yu et al., 2008).

1.2.12.3 Deep Learning

Deep learning is a type of machine learning that employs advanced neural networks to analyze and learn from data (Day and Lee, 2016). These neural networks are sported after the human brain, which comprises millions of neurons. What sets deep learning networks apart is their ability to be utilized in supervised and unsupervised learning scenarios. But deep learning uses neural networks on a large amount of data. Deep learning has exceptional power in learning different patterns in data.

Deep learning includes many networks, including convolutional networks, recurrent neural networks, etc.

Neural networks are widely used in textual data for vector display, sentence classification, sentence modeling, etc. (Zhang et al., 2016).

The greater the number of layers in the neural network, the greater the learning capacity, and more complex problems can be solved. Another very important feature in deep learning is the use of cheap computing in parallel. In deep learning, complex calculations can be done with GPU instead of CPU, and this increases the speed of learning and performing calculations. As you can see in Figure 1.6, the feature selection stage exists in traditional machine learning methods. It is a very time-consuming step that deep learning has been able to eliminate this step and the machine automatically engineers the features. Real applications of deep learning include automatic translation, talking robots and driverless cars, speech recognition, action recognition in video, and emotion recognition and analysis in text. In sentiment analysis with

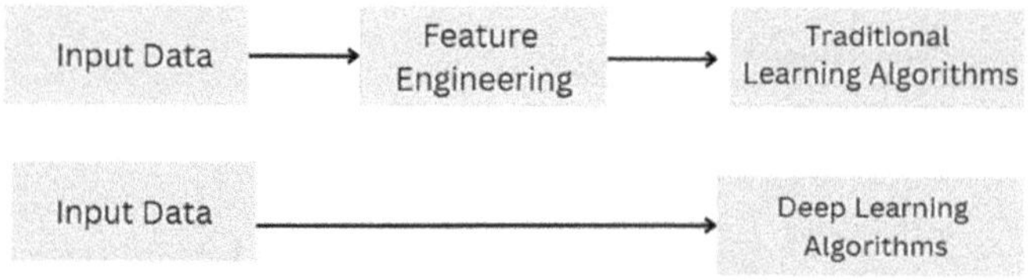

FIGURE 1.6 Traditional learning process compared to deep learning.

deep learning, recurrent neural networks are used, which are many-to-one neural networks. That is, our input is a sequence of words, and the output of the emotion they convey is whether the sentence is positive or negative.

1.2.13 Applications of Sentiment Analysis

With the availability of a huge number of opinions and data in blogs, commenting sites, chat rooms, and social networks, the attention of the academic community and industry was drawn to this field. Sentiment analysis helps service providers understand the mindset of their audience and users and adjust their services according to users' needs.

1.2.13.1 Application of Sentiment Analysis in Business

Among the commercial applications of sentiment analysis, the following can be mentioned:

- Automatic tracking of opinions collected by users and rating of brands, products, and services
- Analyzing the behavior of customers, competitors, and commercial brands
- Observing the general reaction to the changes related to the organization, for example, when presenting a new product, you can analyze the behavior of users and find out their level of satisfaction or dissatisfaction.
- Finding out about the criticisms of users and transferring the problem to the desired department to investigate the problem and fix it

1.2.13.2 Application of Sentiment Analysis in Political Issues

In recent years, sentiment analysis has been used a lot in politics. Among its applications, we can mention the use of sentiment analysis in elections. Social networks are a huge source of opinions, feelings, and criticisms of the people of the society, which can be a very good guide for politicians to observe the needs of the society and plan according to them, and use them for their own benefit in election campaigns.

1.2.13.3 Application of Sentiment Analysis in Recommender Systems

With sentiment analysis, it is possible to learn about the interests of users and act on them for advertising and recommending issues that are of interest to the user, which can be a website, book, article, movie, music, etc. Recommender systems can also be used in political and commercial matters.

Users of digital sales websites usually express their opinions and criticisms about a product after buying it, and these opinions are a very useful database for product manufacturers or its seller's website. One of the most famous and popular of these websites is Amazon. This company also provides its data to researchers for research and analysis of collected opinions, and the results of their research are used to improve the products available on the website or to suggest popular products, etc. Slow.

1.3 RESULTS AND DISCUSSION

1.3.1 Convolutional Network with 64 Filters

The desired convolutional network in the first layer has 64 convolutional filters with sizes of 5 × 5 and a ReLu activation function. After that, we applied a 4 × 4 Maxpooling layer to it. Also, we placed a fully connected layer including 128 neurons whose activation function was ReLu after the Maxpooling layer. To avoid overfitting, we used a dropout rate of 0.2. At the end, we placed a fully connected layer that has two neurons. We also used Categorical cross entropy to measure the network cost and improved the network error rate by using the continuation weight optimizer function.

The results obtained based on the confusion matrix 2 obtained from this model for the test data are shown in Figure 1.7. The ratio of the evaluation criteria on the training data after 100 times when we gave the data to the network was obtained according to Figure 1.7.

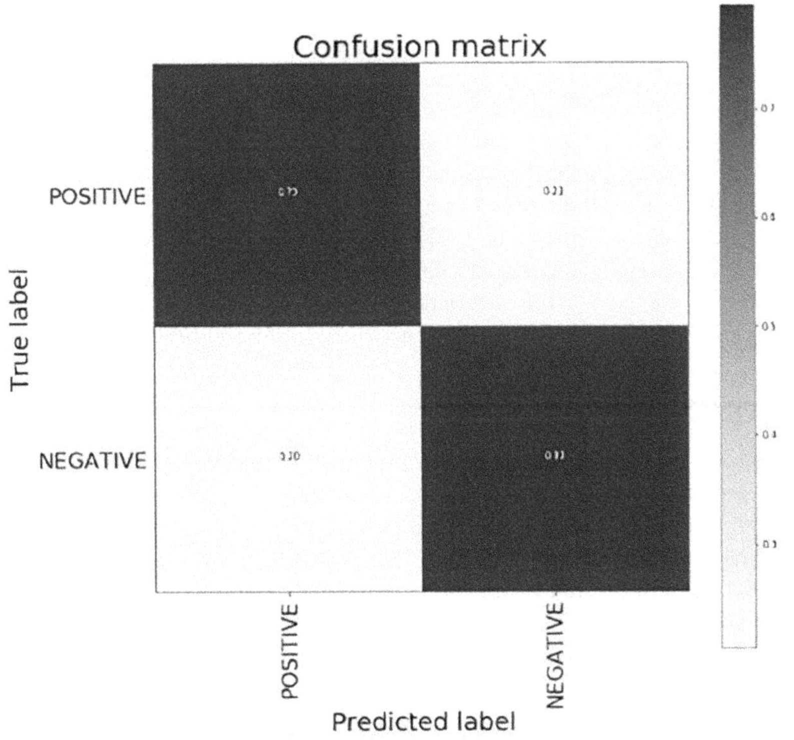

FIGURE 1.7 The ratio of evaluation criteria on the data.

TABLE 1.2
Rate of Tweets by Country

Country	Count
United States	93,423
India	5,330
United Kingdom	8,168
Other	132,164
All	239,094

TABLE 1.3
Analysis of Positive, Negative, and Neutral Comments

Country	Label	Counts	Accuracy
United States	Negative	21,618	25.93%
United States	Neutral	26,851	32.21%
United States	Positive	34,905	41.87%
Grand Total		83,374	100.00%

1.3.2 Basic Information

The research sample was selected and analyzed according to the tweets published in the United States of America, which has the highest rate of tweets among the countries of the world. The population of the United States of America in 2021 is about 329.5 million people, of which about 77.7 million people are active on Twitter. Table 1.2 below shows the rate of tweets by country

As seen in Table 1.2, the United States has the most tweets in the field of Health Care Services among countries with 93,432.

In the next step, the data that was in the field of Health Care Services was extracted, and you can see the number of positive, negative, or neutral tweets in Table 1.3.

1.4 CONCLUSION

Sentiment analysis is one of the most widely used fields in data science and natural language processing. Using the results obtained from sentiment analysis, significant progress can be made in many scientific, social, and commercial fields. Over the years, several approaches have been developed for social media data sentiment analysis. The sentiment analysis process can be complex and time-consuming due to the large volume of data and the need for high accuracy. There are several methods for sentiment analysis, which can be classified into two categories. Methods based on data vocabulary and methods based on machine learning. In recent studies, more machine learning algorithms have been used to categorize texts. Machine learning is done using two approaches: supervised learning and unsupervised learning. In both methods, relatively large datasets are needed, and some researchers try hard to prepare these datasets to make them available to researchers of other sciences. In the current research, the goal was to analyze the sentiment of the texts available on the social network, and for this purpose, the text data available on Twitter was used. Twitter Sentiment Analysis is a valuable and convenient tool for tracking sentiment about news and people's opinions about Health Care Services on Twitter. As mentioned, sentiment analysis or opinion polling are processes that receive, extract, and categorize opinions, emotions, and feelings about a topic, which can be anything, including a product, a person, or a service. The opinions used in this matter are direct and can be categorized as +ve, −ve, or neutral based on the document, sentence, or word and feature levels. Sentiment analysis during health care service is still open and contains many exciting topics that use advanced machine learning and deep learning methods.

This research seeks to analyze the data of the Twitter social network by using the published tweets related to Health Care Services in order to analyze the positive, negative, and neutral opinions of the users of this field by using the technique of sentiment analysis in the fields of deep learning and machine learning. The implication of this study is also evident from the recent situation of the Health Care Service, as information expressed through social media has influenced public sentiment (Depoux et al., 2020). Further, by using machine algorithms, the research has sought to maximize the prediction accuracy of new data.

The method used is classification by deep learning algorithms in two and three classes. We implemented the convolutional network with 64, 128, and 256 filters, as well as the short-term, long-term memory network and the long-short-term memory hybrid model with the 64-filter convolutional network. For each model, standard evaluation criteria in sentiment analysis problems include accuracy. In this study, precision, recall, and f-criterion are calculated. In the binary classification, good results were obtained, and in the long-term, short-term memory model, we achieved an accuracy of 0.85, which is considered a good and valuable result. In the rest of the models, we achieved accuracy above 0.80%, which is generally acceptable when working with the data. In the three-class classification, the evaluation criteria were lower than the binary classification, and the reason for this could be the smallness of the dataset. As the number of categories increases, the details to be learned by the system increase, so more learning data is needed to achieve good results. To improve the results, the Authors in this study once again used the K-Fold validation method to validate the data; as we expected, the results improved a lot, and in the best model, which was the long-short-term memory network model, we achieved an accuracy of 0.94.

The research sample was selected and analyzed according to the tweets published in the United States of America, which has the highest rate of tweets among the world's countries. In the next step, the data in the Health Care Service field was extracted, and the number of positive, negative, or neutral comments on the tweets was examined. According to the findings, people in the United States of America had 25.93% negative opinions, 32.21% neutral opinions, and 41.87% positive opinions in their tweets on Twitter regarding the news of Health Care Services. Considering the analysis of users' opinions and feelings about the news and measures taken in the field of Health Care Service can be used for policy-making and macro decisions of the country, then the results obtained by using the analysis of the feelings of American users. The results found on Twitter indicate that the polarity of users' opinions and feelings was more positive, so policies should be made in this direction. Also, this data about Health Care Services shows us how people, government organizations, and media agencies spread information on social media.

1.4.1 Future Offers

Among the suggestions for future studies, the following can be mentioned:

- It is suggested that language models be used in future works to check the accuracy of sentiment analysis. The purpose of the linguistic model is to teach the system to predict the next data based on the input data. The work can be clearly seen in the Google search engine today.
- It is also possible to develop the existing methods in such a way that instead of bipolar classification, it is classified in a multi-polar way; that is, the intensity of the positive or negative opinion of an opinion can also be determined, and the messages are, for example, divided into five groups. Categorized as negative, negative, neutral, positive, and very positive or that in addition to being positive and negative, emotional states in the text such as surprise, happiness, sadness, or hatred can be recognized. For this purpose, either a dictionary should be compiled with explanations and categories of emotional states, or these states or related words should be taught to the system with supervised machine learning methods.
- Social network messages contain emoticons that can convey different concepts, such as happiness, sadness, anger, and surprise. These emoticons can contain precious messages for sentiment analysis. It is suggested that sentiment analysis be done considering these emoticons in future works.

REFERENCES

Abbasi, F., Sohrabi, B., Manian, A., and Khadior, A. (2016). Presenting a model to categorize the sensitivities of book buyers using a hybrid approach. *Smart Business Management Studies*, 6(21), 65–92.

Aflakparast, M., de Gunst, M., and vanWieringen, W. (2020). Analysis of Twitter data with the Bayesian fused graphical lasso. *PLoS One*, 15, e0235596.

Alamoodi, A. H., Zaidan, B. B., Zaidan, A. A., Albahri, O. S., Mohammed, K. I., Malik, R. Q., Almahdi, E. M., Chyad, M. A., Tareq, Z., Albahri, A. S., and Hameed, H. (2021). Sentiment analysis and its applications in fighting COVID-19 and infectious diseases: A systematic review. *Expert Systems with Applications*, 167, 114155.

Al-Daihani, S. M. and Abrahams, A. (2016). A text mining analysis of academic libraries' tweets. *The Journal of Academic Librarianship*, 42(2), 135–143.

Alsaeedi, A. and Khan, M. Z. (2019). A study on sentiment analysis techniques of Twitter data. *International Journal of Advanced Computer Science and Applications*, 10(2), 361–374.

Barreto, S., Moura, R., Carvalho, J., Paes, A., and Plastino, A. (2021). Sentiment analysis in tweets: An assessment study from classical to modern text representation models. *arXiv preprint arXiv:2105.14373.*

Bhanuse, S. S., Kamble, S. D., and Kakde, S. M. (2016). Text mining using metadata for generation of side information. *Procedia Computer Science*, 78, 807–814. doi: 10.1016/j.procs.2016.02.061

Boyd, D. M. and Ellison N. B. (2007). Social network sites: Definition, history, and scholarship. *Journal of Computer-Mediated Communication*, 13 (1), 210–230. doi: 10.1111/j.1083-6101.2007.00393.x

Cambria, E. and Hussain, A. (2015). *Sentic Computing: A Common-Sense-Based Framework for Concept-Level Sentiment Analysis*. Cham: Springer.

Carvalho, J. and Plastino, A. (2021). On the evaluation and combination of state-of-the-art features in Twitter sentiment analysis. *Artificial Intelligence Review*, 54(3), 1887–1936.

Chen, M. S., Han, J., and Yu, P. S. (1996). Data mining: An overview from a database perspective. *IEEE Transactionson Knowledge and Data Engineering*, 8(6), 866–883.

Depoux, A., Martin, S., Karafillakis, E., Preet, R., Wilder-Smith, A., and Larson, H. (2020). The pandemic of social media panic travels faster than the COVID-19 outbreak. *Journal of Travel Medicine*, 27, taaa031.

Hawalah, A. and Fasli, M. (2015). Dynamic user profiles for web personalization. *Expert Systems with Applications*, 42, 2547–2569.

Injadat, M. N., Salo, F., and Nassif, A. B. (2016). Data mining techniques in social media: A survey, *Neurocomputing*, 214, 654–670. doi: 10.1016/j.neucom.2016.06.045

Ji, X., Chun, S. A., & Geller, J. (2016). Knowledge-based tweet classification for disease sentiment monitoring. *Sentiment Analysis and Ontology Engineering: An Environment of Computational Intelligence*, 425–454.

Jiang, Z., Bai, W., and Bin, W. (2014). Social network users clustering based on multivariate time series of motional behavior. *The Journal of China Universities of Posts and Telecommunications*, 21(2), 21–31. www.sciencedirect.com/science/journal/10058885

Kang, J. and Lee, H. (2017). Modeling user interest in social media using news media and Wikipedia. *Information Systems,* 65, 52–64.

Khobzi, H. and Teimourpour, B. (2015). LCP segmentation: A framework for evaluation of user engagement in online social networks. *Computers in Human Behavior*, 50, 101–107.

Kim, K. S. and Sin, S. C. J. (2016). Use and evaluation of information from social media in the academic context: Analysis of gap between students and librarians. *The Journal of Academic Librarianship,* 42, 74–82. doi: 10.1016/j.acalib.2015.11.001

Lazard, A. J., Scheinfeld, E., Bernhardt, J. M., Wilcox, G. B., and Suran, M. (2015). Detecting themes of public concern: A text mining analysis of the Centers for Disease Control and Prevention's Ebola live Twitter chat. *American Journal of Infection Control*, 1, 1–3. doi: 10.1016/j.ajic.2015.05.025

Liu, B. (2012). *Sentiment Analysis and Opinion Mining (Synthesis Lectures on Human Language Technologies)* (p. 168). Williston, ND: Morgan & Claypool Publishers.

Liu, B. (2015). *Sentiment Analysis: Mining Opinions, Sentiments, and Emotions.* Cambridge University Press, CRC Press.

Manguri, K. H., Ramadhan, R. N., and Amin, P. R. M. (2020). Twitter sentiment analysis on worldwide COVID-19 outbreaks. *Kurdistan Journal of Applied Research*, 5(3), 54–65.

Mohammadi, A., Yazdian-Dehkordi, M., and Nematbakhsh, M. A. (2019). Recognition of implicit features using the syntactic rules of the Persian language and attribute clustering. *Journal of Electrical Engineering of Tabriz University*, 93(3), 1395–1404.

Nair, V. and Hinton, G. E. (2020). Rectified linear units improve restricted Boltzmann machines. In *Proceedings of the 27th International Conference on Machine Learning (ICML-10)*, Canada (pp. 807–814).

Nielsen, F. Å. (2011). A new ANEW: Evaluation of a word list for sentiment analysis in microblogs. In *Proceedings of the ESWC2011 Workshop on 'Making Sense of Microposts': Big Things Come in Small Packages*, Heraklion, Crete, Greece (p. 26).

Niknam, F. and NikNafs, A. (2015). Improving text mining methods in the application of market forecasting using prototype selection algorithms. *Journal of Information Technology Management*, 8(2), 415–434.

Ortigosa, A., Carro, R. M., and Quiroga, J. I. (2014). Predicting user personality by mining social interactions in Facebook. *Journal of Computer and System Sciences*, 80(1), 57–71.

Pandey, A., Rajpoor, D., and Saraswat, M. (2017). Twitter sentiment analysis using hybrid cuckoo search method. *Information Processing and Management*, 53(4), 779–764. doi: 10.1016/j.ipm.2017.02.004

Pham, D. -H. and Le, A. -C. (2018). Learning multiple layers of knowledge representation for aspect-based sentiment analysis. *Data & Knowledge Engineering*, 114, 26–39.

Pourgholam Ali, F., Kahani, M., and Asgarian, E. (2019). Using big data technology for opinion research. *Scientific Journal of Soft Computing*, 9(1), 26–39.

Singh, C., Imam, T., Wibowo, S., and Grandhi, S. (2022). A deep learning approach for sentiment analysis of COVID-19 reviews. *Applied Sciences*, 12(8), 3709.

Singh, C., Wibowo, S., and Grandhi, S. (2020). An integrated non-linear deep learning method for sentiment classification of online reviews. In *Advances in Natural Computation, Fuzzy Systems and Knowledge Discovery* (pp. 1–8), Meng, H., Lei, T., Li, M., Li, K., Xiong, N., Wang, L., Eds. Cham: Springer.

Sohrabi, B., Raisi Vanani, I., Talebian, M. (2015). Presenting a model for analyzing the behavior of social network users using data mining methods: A social network in Iran. *Organizational Resource Management Research*, 6(4), 83–106.

Tsiotsou, R. H. (2015). The role of social and parasocial relationships on social networking sites loyalty. *Computers in Human Behavior*, 48, 401–414.

van Dam, J. M., and van de Velden, M.(2014). Online profiling and clustering of Facebook users. *Decision Support Systems*. doi: 10.1016/j.dss.2014.12.001

Wang, Y., Wang, M., and Xu, W. (2018). A sentiment-enhanced hybrid recommender system for movie recommendation: An extensive data analytics framework. *Wireless Communications and Mobile Computing* 2018(1), 8263704.

Yu, B., Xu, Z. B., and Li, C. H. (2008). Latent semantic analysis for text categorization using neural network. *Knowledge-Based Systems*, 21(8), 900–904.

Zhao, P. and Zhang, C.O. (2011). A new clustering method and its application in social networks. *Pattern Recognition Letters*, 32, 2109–2118.

2 Non-Sorted Genetic Algorithm and Logistic Regression (NSGA-LR) for Prediction of Heart Diseases

Shahzad Latif, Sajjad A. Ghauri, Aizhar Ali, and Mariyum Munir

2.1 INTRODUCTION

Heart disease and cancer are responsible for 70% of all deaths, equivalent to 41 million people around the globe [1]. These two health issues are the most significant challenges faced by the world, where CVD is the leading death-taking and cardiac disease to cover glitches of the heart [2]. Constriction and blockage of blood vessels can result in heart disease and eventually lead to a heart attack. There are several factors, which include diabetes, smoking, high blood pressure, high blood cholesterol, and alcohol consumption, that can trigger this illness [3]. The symptoms of a heart attack may differ between men and women. Men usually experience chest pain, while women may experience chest pain, discomfort, shortness of breath, nausea, and extreme fatigue. Symptoms of intrinsic coronary illness may include excessive sweating, high levels of fatigue, rapid heartbeat, shortness of breath, chest pain, a blue tint to the skin, and clubbed fingernails [4].

The National Institute of Health and the American Heart Association publish annual cardiovascular risk factors, heart disease, and stroke statistics [5]. There are various medical conditions and lifestyle choices that can lead to heart disease, including:

1. Excessive alcohol consumption
2. Inactivity on the physical level
3. Unhealthy eating habits
4. Diabetes, Obesity, and Overweight

Coronary angiography (CHD) is a highly accurate and reliable invasive procedure to diagnose coronary heart disease. The current system is inadequate when detecting CHD during the annual assessment. Echocardiography and

DOI: 10.1201/9781003469896-2

Electrocardiogram are non-invasive techniques, but they are only sometimes reliable in terms of accuracy. It is essential to prioritize using non-invasive methods to identify CHD [6].

In clinical cardiology, machine learning has been demonstrated as a successful strategy for predicting heart disease patients. By implementing intelligent systems as decision support systems in hospitals, medical professionals can benefit from an additional viewpoint on specific diseases and conditions. This can enhance their ability to make informed decisions and provide optimal care to their patients. Coronary disease is a critical issue that demands immediate attention. The high mortality rates are linked to delayed clinical treatment and insufficient early detection. The decision tree techniques, Naive Bayes, neural networks, ANN, logistic regression, and support vector machines are traditional machine learning techniques for classification problems. The application of these methodologies led to enhanced outcomes in heart disease prediction, resulting in improved performance. Additionally, ensemble machine-learning approaches were employed to enhance the effectiveness of traditional machine-learning models, further elevating the accuracy of heart disease prediction [7].

In Ref. [8], the study explores ensemble classification to enhance weak algorithms accuracy by combining multiple classifiers. Through experiments on a heart disease dataset, the research demonstrates that ensemble techniques like bagging and boosting effectively improve prediction accuracy. Additionally, feature selection further enhances accuracy, showcasing this approach's utility in early-stage disease prediction. In Ref. [9], authors have identified the key characteristics and machine learning classification methods that can enhance the accuracy of predicting coronary heart disease. The brute force was used as a feature selection approach, identifying nine segments from the 13 parts Cleveland dataset of UCI. Authors of Ref. [10] introduced the Genetic Algorithm (GA) approach for identifying the crucial features related to heart conditions. They applied GA to the Cleveland UCI dataset and selected seven essential features for predicting heart disease.

In Ref. [11], a method was developed for coronary illness diagnosis using unsupervised and supervised machine learning techniques. The proposed method for predicting heart disease involves using the self-organizing map technique to select 11 out of 13 features from the UCI dataset of Statlog and Cleveland. The incremental principal component analysis is utilized to streamline computations by reducing the dimensions of the data. Two imputation techniques, K Nearest Neighbor and HotDeck, fill in missing values. Finally, the incremental fuzzy support vector machine is used for heart disease classification and shows significant improvement.

However, the proposed classifiers still need to meet satisfactory and promising accuracy results. Rather than training one classifier, multiple classifiers can be combined to achieve robust and efficient results. It has been shown that hybrid models also work well in other domains. Improving accuracy and selecting significant features of heart disease remains an open research challenge.

The early prediction of heart attacks can potentially mitigate the fatality risk. Various machine-learning approaches are leveraged for this purpose. The accuracy of predicting heart attacks poses a challenge, as it is a non-convex problem with NP-hard characteristics [12]. In response to this challenge, NSGA-LR is introduced as a solution to enhance the accuracy of heart attack prediction. Furthermore, a hybrid dataset encompassing a comprehensive array of heart disease features addresses this concern.

2.1.1 Contribution of the Article

The main contributions of the paper are as follows:

1. The paper conducts a comprehensive study and analysis of various machine learning algorithms commonly used for early prediction of heart attacks. This analysis helps understand the strengths and weaknesses of different algorithms in this specific application domain.
2. The paper proposes a novel NSGA-LR (Non-Sorting Genetic Algorithm Logistic Regression Algorithm) designed for early heart attack prediction. NSGA-LR combines the principles of genetic algorithms and logistic regression to enhance the accuracy and efficiency of prediction. The algorithm aims to address the limitations of existing methods and provide improved performance.

The paper compares the performance of the proposed algorithms commonly used in heart attack prediction. The paper also includes a comparison with other under-studied algorithms that may have the potential for early heart attack prediction. This comparative analysis helps evaluate the effectiveness and superiority of the NSGA-LR algorithm in terms of accuracy, computational efficiency, and other relevant performance metrics.

2.1.2 Organization of the Article

The article's structure is as follows: Section 2.2 presents the existing work on heart diseases, and approximately all the machine learning algorithms are discussed with various features. The proposed framework is comprehensively presented in Section 2.3 with feature selection, feature scaling, Logistic regression, Stacking, and Genetic algorithm. Section 2.4 presents the experimental setup with a detailed discussion of the simulation results with a comparative analysis. The article is concluded at the end with some future directions in Section 2.5.

2.2 RELATED WORK

The critical analysis includes an overview of the research that has been done on heart disease prediction. As shown above, in Table 2.1, many studies have been conducted to better predict heart disease by highlighting the key features of this disease. The techniques used in heart disease prediction, their weakness, and their strengths are also shown in Table 2.1. The classifiers proposed so far still do not meet satisfying and promising results in accuracy. Unlike training a single classifier, multiple classifiers can be combined to produce robust and efficient results. The hybrid models are showing promising results in other domains. Still, heart disease's significant feature selection and accuracy improvement is an open research challenge.

TABLE 2.1
Review of Existing Techniques

Reference	Methodology	Strength	Accuracy/Limitation
[13]	Hybrid random forest linear model	High accuracy	Lacking in precision, F-measure, sensitivity
[14]	Improved SVM-RBF	Better accuracy with hyperparameters	Not suitable for large dataset
[15]	Floating window width adaptive size for feature elimination	High efficiency	Slow hyper-parameter tunning
[16]	Modified Artificial Plant Optimization (MAPO)	Seven features improved accuracy	89%
[17]	Optimized stacked SVM	Eight optimal features	Low accuracy on non-linearly separable data
[18]	Combination of XGBoost BDSCAN and SMOTE-ENN	Detection and removal of data outliers	Low accuracy
[19]	Random tree model	40 optimal features	Over-fitting issue
[20]	K-NN	–	No feature selection
[21]	Chi-square and PCA	Better performance as compared to raw dataset features	–
[22]	Big data predictive analysis-naive bayes	High accuracy	Not compatible dataset
[23]	ACO-hybrid KNN	9-important features	More time complexity
[24]	Adaptive genetic algorithm with Fuzzy logic	Efficiently processed high dimension noisy data	Less accurate
[25]	PSO-feature selection	Two-tier architecture	Computationally expensive
[26]	Hybrid loin and PSO algorithm	Outperformed	Local minima issue
[27]	Discrete weights	Improved results	No comparison
[28]	PRISM + PGA	–	88%

The evolutionary algorithms demonstrated superior performance in feature selection for the heart disease dataset. These selected features were then utilized in machine learning classification techniques, resulting in improved accuracy in predicting heart disease. While prediction accuracy remains a primary focus, addressing solution complexity could be a key area for future research in heart disease prediction systems.

2.3 PROPOSED MODEL

The proposed methodology will use an open-source or secondary heart disease dataset from the UCI repository of machine learning data sets. After checking the dataset, the following stage is pre-processing and information discretization as data cleaning, transformation, reduction, binning, and attribute selection. After applying every one of these strategies to the dataset, correlation study and feature selection methods will be used. Later, a hybrid ensemble machine learning technique will be applied to the data and compare the results. The proposed system model is shown in Figure 2.1.

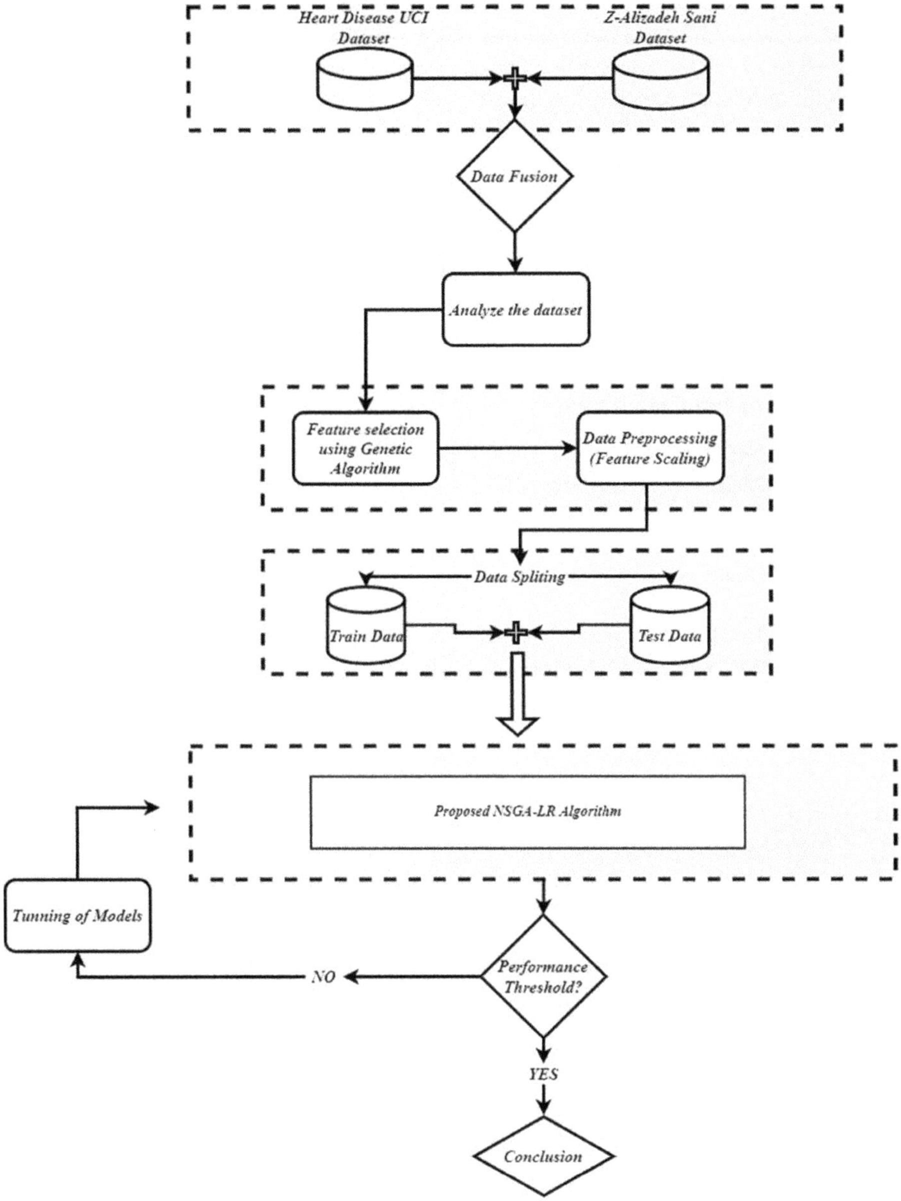

FIGURE 2.1 Proposed system model.

2.3.1 Data-Set Description

The dataset part of the experimental process is the Cleveland heart disease (CHD) dataset from the UCI repository of machine learning datasets [29]. It consists of 303 observations of the heart disease patient with 14 features or attributes like sex, blood sugar, chest pain type, ST-segment slope, blood pressure resting, and age. The target variable is also part of 14 features that define whether a patient has a disease or no disease. Table 2.2 lists the dataset's attributes with the description and values.

The slope is related to exercise and the person's heart rate. The risk of heart disease in the next ten years can be figured out by the doctors by checking the level of the patient's cholesterol. The Chole is the cholesterol level in the patient's blood in mg/dL. The Thal is an essential categorical feature that defines the amount of blood to the different parts of the heart. Exang is an important feature related to exercise and the demand for oxygen to the heart. The narrowed arteries slow down the flow of blood to the heart when the patient exercise, climb stairs, and does physical activity.

TABLE 2.2
Attributes of the CHD Dataset

Sr. No.	Attribute	Description	Value
1	Slope	The slope of the peak exercise segment	1: Up sloping 2: Flat 3: Down sloping
2	Gender	Male/female	1: Male 0: Female
3	Trest bps	Resting blood pressure (mm Hg)	Continuous
4	Cp	Chest pain type	1: Typical angina 2: Atypical angina 3: Non-anginal pain 4: Asymptomatic
5	Chole	Serum cholesterol (mg/dL)	Continuous
6	FBS	Fasting blood sugar	1: ≥120 mg/dL 0: ≤120 mg/dL
7	Thal	Thallium scan	3: Normal 6: Fixed defect 7: Reversible defect
8	Thalach	Maximum heart rate achieved	Continuous
9	Exang	Exercise-induced angina	1: Yes 0: No
10	Old peak	ST depression	Continuous
11	Age	Age in years	Continuous
12	Ca	Number of major vessels colored by fluoroscopy	[1 4]
13	Restecg	Resting electrocardiographic results	0: Normal 1: STT wave abnormality 2: Left ventricular hypertrophy

The other dataset fused with the above dataset of Cleveland is the Z-Alizadeh Sani dataset from the UCI repository of machine learning datasets [30]. It consists of 303 observations of heart disease patients with 56 features or attributes like Exsmoker, Obesity, ejection fraction (EF) in %, etc.

- **Data-set fusion**: The next step is data fusion because most features are mutually exclusive in both datasets. The process data hybridization considers the Cleveland dataset as the primary dataset for disease prediction, and the features not part of this primary dataset are concatenated with it to increase the information for the machine learning model for the sake of prediction. The exclusive features utilized from the dataset of Z-Alizadeh Sani include the current smoker, Ex-smoker, fh, and bp.

The factor of smoking is very crucial in the prediction of heart disease because this feature is directly proportioned to the feature of cholesterol and tree tops. The feature of smoking is not part of the primary dataset of Cleveland, so due to that reason, this feature is included in the other dataset to increase the performance of machine learning models for the prediction of heart disease. Similarly, the other features are also part of the hybrid dataset. The combination of features is performed around the feature axis to increase the features.

2.3.2 Feature Selection and Validation

In the prediction of heart disease, NSGA is used for feature selection. The technique of NSGA performed well in selecting features from a hybrid dataset. The total features are 45 in the dataset, and the dependent variable has a binary output of zero or one that will define patient has a disease or not. The machine learning techniques first run on a complete feature dataset, but the accuracy achieved by these techniques was not very high. The selected features improved the accuracy of algorithms, and the other performance measures also showed significant improvement.

- **Feature scaling**: The concept of feature normalization or scaling is to put all the data set's features in a specific range to boost the machine learning algorithm calculations. In the data pre-processing process, feature scaling is performed on the independent variable of the dataset to achieve better performance. This process has many techniques, including min-max scalar, z-score normalization or standard scalar, and max-abs scalar. Still, in predicting heart disease, the standard scalar is used to normalize the features of heart disease.

The features of the hybrid dataset include body mass index (BMI), blood pressure (BP), fasting blood sugar (PR), fasting blood sugar (FBS), triglyceride (TG), low-density lipoprotein (LDL), high-density lipoprotein (HDL), high blood urea nitrogen (BUN), erythrocyte sedimentation rate (ESR), hemoglobin levels (HB), white blood cell (WBC), lymph is not in the normal range after applying a standard scaler these features also come into the content of zero to one.

2.3.3 Logistic Regression (LR)

Binary classification is the most basic classification problem in machine learning. In machine learning, many algorithms can model the binary dependent variable, and logistic regression is one model that performs well in binary classification problems [31]. Many more complex extensions of logistic regression exist, but the basic logistic regression algorithm models a binary dependent variable using a logistic function. The dependent variable has two levels in a binary logistic regression model.

The logistic function is the sigmoid function $h_\theta(x)$ and the predicted output for the heart disease; 1 means the patient has the disease, and 0 means the patient has no disease. The $h_\theta(x)$ is defined as:

where α is the linear regressor and expressed as:

Where w_o is an intercept, w_i and x_i represent the ith weight and feature of the data set. The i in our dataset is 45 because the dataset contains 45 features. The equation representing the machine learning linear regression technique is similar to

Algorithm 2.1: LR Pseudo Code 1

```
get
while                do
    for i=1:ℑ do
        Calculate Linear Regressor using Eq. (2)
        Calculate Predicted Output using Eq. (1)
        Calculate Combined Cost Function using Eq. (4)
    end
    for Each Feature j in Sample i do
        Optimize Weights
        wj+1 = wj − α[hθ(x^(i)) − y^(i)]xj^(i)
    end
    if wj+1 == wj then
        break;
    end
end
return y,w
```

Initialize x, y, w_0, w_1, w_2, …, w_n logistic regression. Still, the output generated by logistic regression is binary values between (0, 1). The output generated by the logistic regression is not precise (0 or 1).

The β_0 and β_1 are the weights for the linear equation that will generate the actual value output. The β_0 defines the intercept for the training line of the logistic regression, and β_1 is the movement of the training line of the model for better performance. The gradient descent optimizes the weights of the logistic regression model by achieving a global minimum for accurate classification. Initially, the random weights are assigned for each feature after training these weights to get optimized.

The orange line intercepts at 0.5 and the threshold value for the calculation of the output of the model. If the value exceeds the threshold value, the output will be one and vice versa. The mean square error is the cost function of the linear regression, but it becomes a nonconvex function for the logistic regression model and cannot be used as a cost function. If the function is nonconvex, it can be stuck in local minima and unable to achieve the global minima; hence, the convergence of the gradient descent function must be convex.

Gradient descent is used in the optimization of the cost function of the logistic regression algorithm. As shown in Eq. (2.2), the cost function: $\Xi[h_\theta(x),y]$ for both the binary cases described separately and the y is the actual output of the dataset.

The Eq. (2.2) is the combined cost function of both binary values and is expressed as:

$$\Xi\left[h_\theta(x), y\right] = -y\log\left[h_\theta(x)\right] - (1-y)\log\left[h_\theta(x)\right] \tag{2.2}$$

The pseudo-code of the logistic regression model is shown in Algorithm 2.1.

2.3.4 Stacking

In machine learning applications, combining different machine learning models constantly improves the final results, and the combination of machine learning models is called an ensemble. Several techniques and ensemble methods exist in machine learning, and stacking is one technique that combines the characteristics of strong machine learning models to produce efficient and improved results.

Stacking puts layers of models like neural network layers in deep learning, and machine learning models are neurons of layers [32]. It does not consider the output of only 1 model because its architecture shows the models exist in a base layer called the base learner model, which provides its work to the meta-learner for the final improved prediction. The training data used by different models exist in the base layer and generate output. The meta-learner then uses the prediction or output of these models because the meta-learner input is only the base learner model's output rather than training data. The stacking method is shown in Figure 2.2.

2.3.5 Non-Domination Based GA

Charles Darwin's proposed theory of natural evolution is called Darwin's theory, and this theory inspires the genetic algorithm. The natural algorithm selection of individuals takes place for the process of reproduction of the chain of parent-child for the next generation. The characteristics of the parents are inherited by the child for the next generation—the chances of surviving a child increase when the parents have robust features. The same iterative process goes on, and finally, the generation has strong characteristics of individuals. Strong individuals are the favorite for the natural selection of reproduction in genetic algorithms. The Genetic algorithm is divided into five parts or phases [33–35].

- **First phase**: Initialize Population- In the heart disease dataset, 303 patients' data is the initial population. These individuals are the candidates for the problem solution in the GA.
- **Second phase**: Fitness Function- The total patient population is 303, and each patient has 45 features or genes. The objective function of the algorithm needs to be optimized:

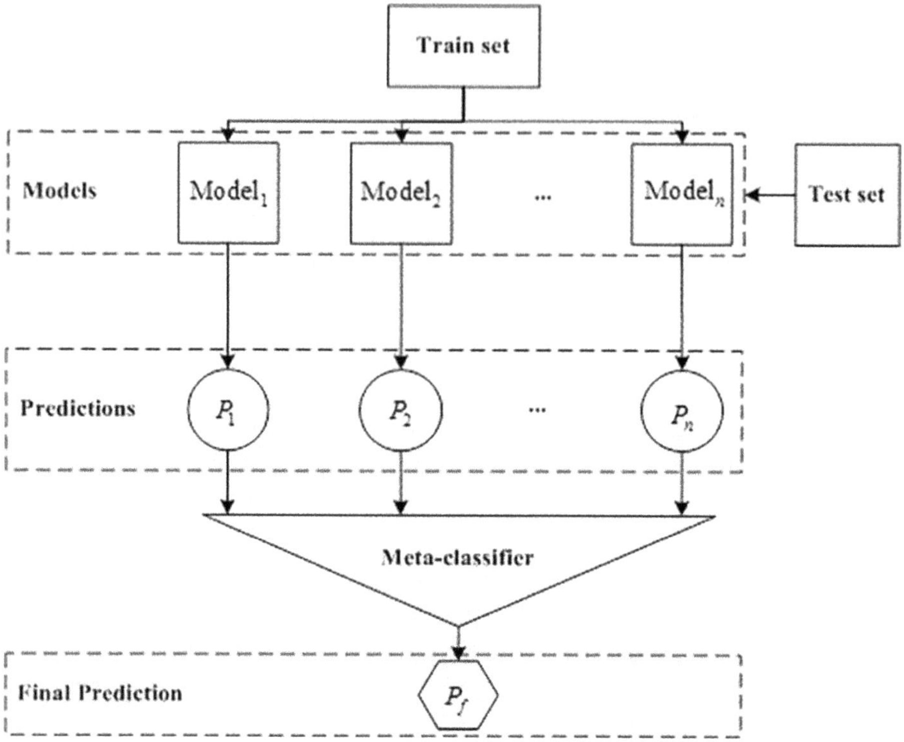

FIGURE 2.2 AI report from 2020 to 2030.

where τ is the total no. of features and X_i is the ith feature vector.

- **Third phase**: Generation Selection- The selection involves picking a strong individual for the upcoming generation. There are many types of selection in GA, including Roulette Wheel Selection, Rank Selection, Tournament Selection, and Boltzmann Selection. In this research work, Roulette Wheel Selection is used for the upcoming generation to predict heart disease.
- **Fourth phase**: Crossover- The most critical phase of the GA is the crossover phase because it is the step where the parents' genes exchange together based on the crossover rate. There are many types of crossovers in GA, including one-point crossover, two-point crossover, order crossover, and cycle cross-over. The two-point crossover was used at 0.76 in the heart disease prediction.
- **Last phase**: Mutation- Controls the chromosome genetic diversity of the next generation.

2.3.6 Evaluation Metrics

Many researchers utilize performance metrics, including accuracy, precision, recall, and F-score, to analyze and calculate the model's accomplishment. The accuracy is measured using Eq. (2.3). Precision is the proportion of correctly predicted positive observations to the total number of expected positive observations and is calculated using Eq. (2.4). The Recall or Sensitivity is shown in Eq. (2.5). The recall is the proportion of correctly anticipated positive observations to all the actual class observations. The F.Score is shown in Eq. (2.6). The F.Score is a total weighted Precision and Recall standard.

$$\text{Accuracy} = \frac{t_p + t_n}{t_p + t_n + f_p + f_n} \tag{2.3}$$

$$\text{Precision} = \frac{t_p}{t_p + f_p} \tag{2.4}$$

$$\text{Re call} = \frac{t_p}{t_p + f_n} \tag{2.5}$$

$$F.\text{Score} = \frac{2 \times \text{Precision} \times \text{Recall}}{\text{Precision} + \text{Recall}} \tag{2.6}$$

where t_p and t_n are the actual numbers of positive and negative examples. f_p and f_n are the wrong predicted positive and negative examples.

2.4 SIMULATION RESULTS

2.4.1 Experimental Setup

The system's specifications are Windows 10 OS with a CPU of 3.20 GHz and 16 GHz of RAM. The proposed model comprises several pieces, each trained on an NVIDIA TITANX GPU. The Jupyter Notebook [36] is used in this research due to its interactive web-based user interface. It lets you share your data analysis, visualization, and machine-learning code as a document. This integrated development environment is part of Anaconda software, which is also open-source and contains all the packages and libraries required for data science and machine learning problems. Python 3 is used due to its high-level programming nature and several libraries available for machine learning and data visualization, including Seaborn [37], Matplotlib [38], and Sciki-learn [39].

Alizadeh Sani dataset was imported using the Pandas Python library for data preprocessing and analysis. These two datasets were concatenated to perform data fusion, resulting in a combined data frame featuring 45 heart disease-related features and one target variable. The number of observations remained consistent at 303.

Subsequently, a genetic algorithm was applied to select relevant features, following which the selected features were scaled for efficient performance of machine learning algorithms. The scaled dataset was then split into training and testing sets using the Scikit-learn library. The training involved 80% of the data, while the remaining 20% was utilized for testing the machine learning models' performance and identifying the most effective one for heart disease prediction.

The proposed NSGA-LR method's performance was compared against that of stochastic gradient descent (SGD), Knearest neighbor (KNN), and Naive Bayes (NB) algorithms for heart disease prediction. Evaluation metrics included accuracy, precision, recall, and F-measure. As depicted in Figure 2.3, the proposed NSGA-LR algorithm outperformed the existing algorithms across all metrics. Notably, Naive Bayes exhibited poor accuracy on the specific heart disease dataset. The proposed NSGA-LR achieved an accuracy of 91.80%, surpassing SGD, KNN, and NB with 90.16%, 78.69%, and 55.74%, respectively.

Figure 2.3 reveals that the technique of Naive Bayes and the lazy learner KNN are achieving low accuracy on the fused dataset (Figure 2.4).

The Stochastic Gradient Descent is also achieving an accuracy of 90% but is still behind the proposed NSGA-LR model in precision, recall, and F score. It is the second-best model of experimental study. The technique of SVM is the third best technique according to an experimental study for heart disease prediction. The comparison of the accuracy of existing machine-learning techniques for heart disease prediction with the proposed method of NSGA-LR is shown in Figure 2.3. The NSGA-LR achieves the highest accuracy of 91.80% (Figures 2.5 and 2.6).

The performance of thirteen machine learning models is compared to the hybrid heart disease dataset. Among these models, the NSGA-LR model achieves better accuracy than other models because NSGA is the algorithm that produces the optimal features using the global search capability by mutation and crossover probabilities.

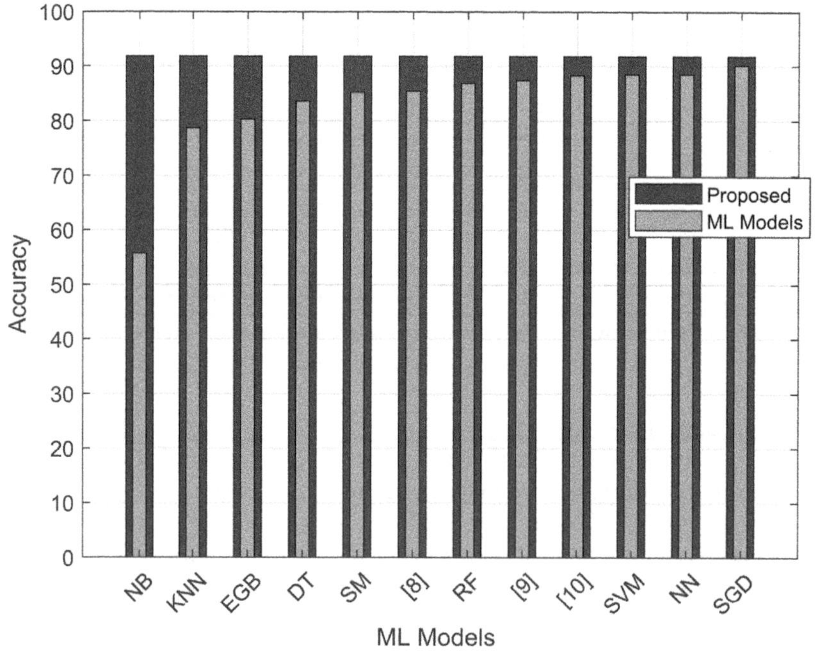

FIGURE 2.3 Accuracy of NSGA-LR with other ML techniques.

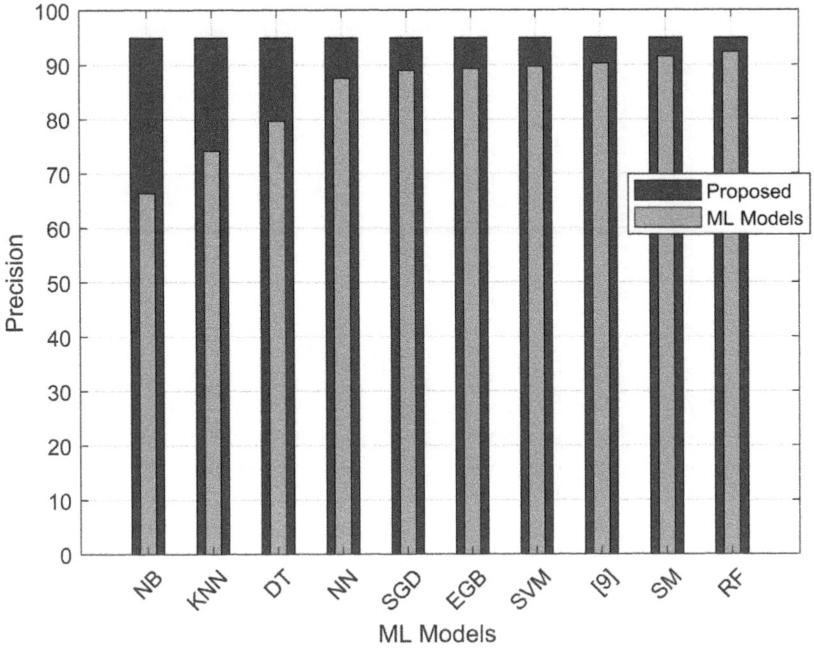

FIGURE 2.4 Precision of NSGA-LR with other ML techniques.

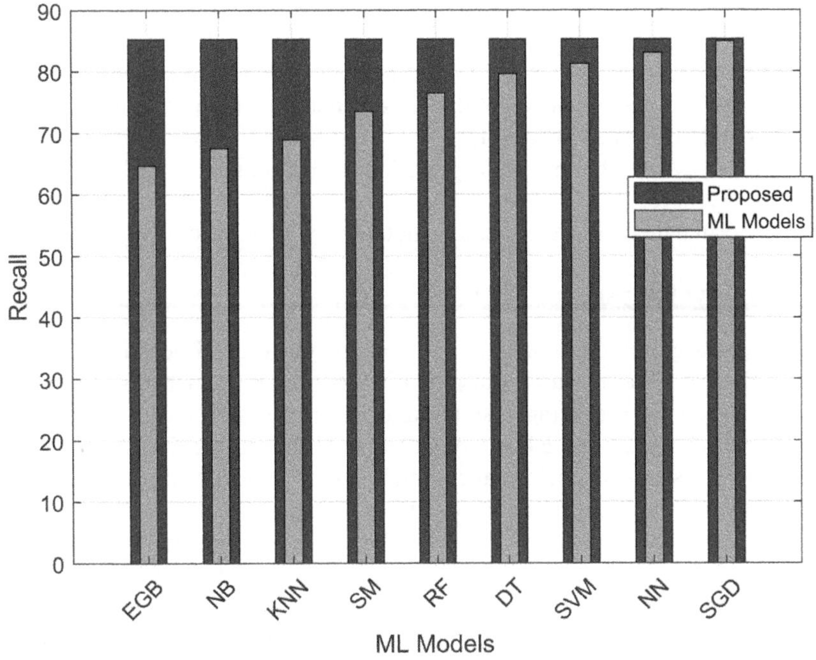

FIGURE 2.5 Recall of NSGA-LR with other ML techniques.

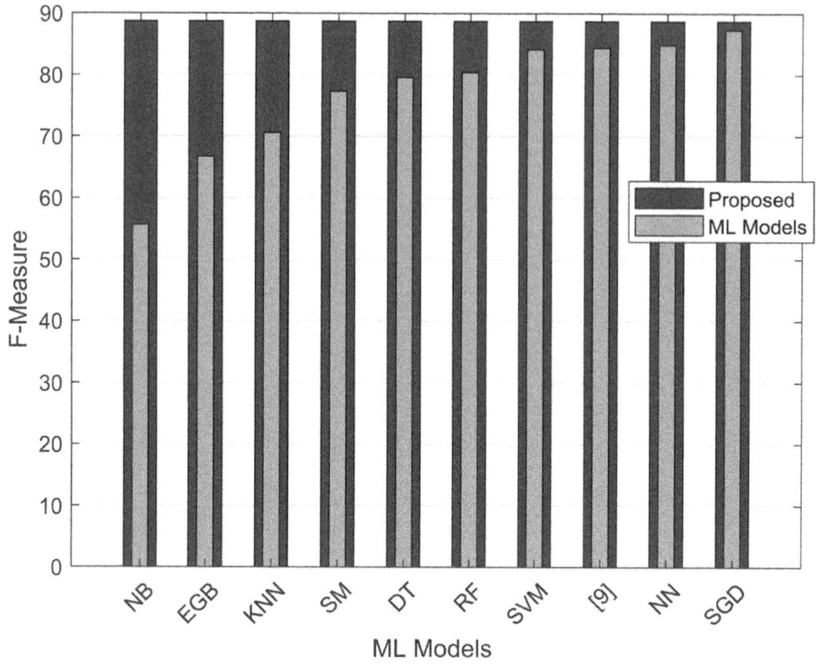

FIGURE 2.6 F-measure of NSGA-LR with other ML techniques.

The LR model maps the linear output into the probability for binary classification of heart methods, including [8–10], but it is also a critical evaluation parameter. In Figure 2.5, the recall score of NSGA-LR was compared with other machine-learning techniques and performed efficiently.

The NSGA-LR exhibits superior precision, as demonstrated in Figures 2.4 and 2.5, with an F.Score.

The performance measure of recall is not discussed in the existing Figure 2.6.

2.5 CONCLUSION

The heart disease prediction model's high accuracy is crucial because it is a severe and fatal disease. The research presented in this paper contributes to early heart attack prediction by providing insights into meta-heuristic and machine-learning based hybrid approach, coined as NSGA-LR, to enhance prediction accuracy, and demonstrate its superior performance compared to other established algorithms. The findings of this research are promising in terms of accuracy; which can guide future studies and advancements in developing more accurate and reliable methods for early detection of heart attacks, ultimately leading to better healthcare outcomes for patients. In the future, combining logistic regression with other metaheuristics algorithms could yield better outcomes. Moreover, feature selection on the hybrid dataset may reveal crucial attributes for future studies. However, in the near future, eAntHocNet can be used to enhance lifetime [40]. This work serves as a valuable resource for researchers [41]. Expanding the comparative analysis with machine learning methods could improve cardiovascular disease prediction further.

REFERENCES

1. Roser, M., and H. Ritchie. "*Causes of Death.*" Our World in Data (2018).
2. Jackson, William M., Matthew Monteleone, An Kim, and Riva Ko. "Memory problems in children with congenital heart disease: A narrative review." *Journal of Neurosurgical Anesthesiology* 35, no. 1 (2023): 136–141.
3. Dougherty, Scott, Emmy Okello, Jeremiah Mwangi, and Raman Krishna Kumar. "Rheumatic heart disease: JACC focus seminar 2/4." *Journal of the American College of Cardiology* 81, no. 1 (2023): 81–94.
4. Zhang, Qin, Zhiwei Guo, Yanyan Zhu, Pandi Vijayakumar, Aniello Castiglione, and Brij B. Gupta. "A deep learning-based fast fake news detection model for cyber-physical social services." *Pattern Recognition Letters* 168 (2023): 31–38.
5. Johnson, Pamela T., Sarah J. Conway, Scott A. Berkowitz, Armin Arbab-Zadeh, Lee H. Riley, Nisha Gilotra, Nestoras N. Mathioudakis, Leonard Feldman, and Amit K. Pahwa. "Transforming health care from volume to value: A health system implementation road map." *The American Journal of Medicine* 136, no. 8 (2023): 763–767.
6. Mohapatra, Subasish, Sushree Maneesha, Subhadarshini Mohanty, Prashanta Kumar Patra, Sourav Kumar Bhoi, Kshira Sagar Sahoo, and Amir H. Gandomi. "A stacking classifiers model for detecting heart irregularities and predicting cardiovascular disease." *Healthcare Analytics* 3 (2023): 100133.
7. Hajiarbabi, Mohammadreza. "Heart disease detection using machine learning methods: A comprehensive narrative review." *Journal of Medical Artificial Intelligence* 7 (2024).
8. Latha, C. Beulah Christalin, and S. Carolin Jeeva. "Improving the accuracy of prediction of heart disease risk based on ensemble classification techniques." *Informatics in Medicine Unlocked* 16 (2019): 100203.
9. Amin, Mohammad Shafenoor, Yin Kia Chiam, and Kasturi Dewi Varathan. "Identification of significant features and data mining techniques in predicting heart disease." *Telematics and Informatics* 36 (2019): 82–93.
10. Gokulnath, Chandra Babu, and S. P. Shantharajah. "An optimized feature selection based on genetic approach and support vector machine for heart disease." *Cluster Computing* 22 (2019): 14777–14787.
11. Nilashi, Mehrbakhsh, Hossein Ahmadi, Azizah Abdul Manaf, Tarik A. Rashid, Sarminah Samad, Leila Shahmoradi, Nahla Aljojo, and Elnaz Akbari. "Coronary heart disease diagnosis through self-organizing map and fuzzy support vector machine with incremental updates." *International Journal of Fuzzy Systems* 22 (2020): 1376–1388.
12. Burse, Rashmi, and Rajesh Wadhvani. "Comparative analysis of various regularization techniques in the prediction of heart diseases." In *2017 International Conference on Inventive Computing and Informatics (ICICI)*, pp. 356–361. IEEE, 2017.
13. Mohan, Senthilkumar, Chandrasegar Thirumalai, and Gautam Srivastava. "Effective heart disease prediction using hybrid machine learning techniques." *IEEE Access* 7 (2019): 81542–81554.
14. Harimoorthy, Karthikeyan, and Menakadevi Thangavelu. "Retracted article: Multi-disease prediction model using improved SVM-radial bias technique in healthcare monitoring system." *Journal of Ambient Intelligence and Humanized Computing* 12, no. 3 (2021): 3715–3723.

15. Javeed, Ashir, Sanam Shahla Rizvi, Shijie Zhou, Rabia Riaz, Shafqat Ullah Khan, and Se Jin Kwon. "Heart risk failure prediction using a novel feature selection method for feature refinement and neural network for classification." *Mobile Information Systems* 2020, no. 1 (2020): 8843115.
16. Faustini, Pedro Henrique Arruda, and Thiago Ferreira Covoes. "Fake news detection in multiple platforms and languages." *Expert Systems with Applications* 158 (2020): 113503.
17. Ali, Liaqat, Awais Niamat, Javed Ali Khan, Noorbakhsh Amiri Golilarz, Xiong Xingzhong, Adeeb Noor, Redhwan Nour, and Syed Ahmad Chan Bukhari. "An optimized stacked support vector machines based expert system for the effective prediction of heart failure." IEEE Access 7 (2019): 54007–54014.
18. Fitriyani, Norma Latif, Muhammad Syafrudin, Ganjar Alfian, and Jongtae Rhee. "HDPM: An effective heart disease prediction model for a clinical decision support system." IEEE Access 8 (2020): 133034–133050.
19. Joloudari, Javad Hassannataj, Edris Hassannataj Joloudari, Hamid Saadatfar, Mohammad Ghasemigol, Seyyed Mohammad Razavi, Amir Mosavi, Narjes Nabipour, Shahaboddin Shamshirband, and Laszlo Nadai. "Coronary artery disease diagnosis; ranking the significant features using a random trees model." International Journal of Environmental Research and Public Health 17, no. 3 (2020): 731.
20. Shah, Devansh, Samir Patel, and Santosh Kumar Bharti. "Heart disease prediction using machine learning techniques." SN Computer Science 1, no. 6 (2020): 345.
21. Gárate-Escamila, Anna Karen, Amir Hajjam El Hassani, and Emmanuel Andrès. "Classification models for heart disease prediction using feature selection and PCA." Informatics in Medicine Unlocked 19 (2020): 100330.
22. Venkatesh, R., C. Balasubramanian, and Madasamy Kaliappan. "Development of big data predictive analytics model for disease prediction using machine learning technique." Journal of Medical Systems 43, no. 8 (2019): 272.
23. Yuan, Chunyuan, Qianwen Ma, Wei Zhou, Jizhong Han, and Songlin Hu. "Early detection of fake news by utilizing the credibility of news, publishers, and users based on weakly supervised learning." *arXiv preprint arXiv:2012.04233* (2020).
24. Reddy, G. Thippa, M. Praveen Kumar Reddy, Kuruva Lakshmanna, Dharmendra Singh Rajput, Rajesh Kaluri, and Gautam Srivastava. "Hybrid genetic algorithm and a fuzzy logic classifier for heart disease diagnosis." Evolutionary Intelligence 13 (2020): 185–196.
25. Tama, Bayu Adhi, Sun Im, and Seungchul Lee. "Improving an intelligent detection system for coronary heart disease using a two-tier classifier ensemble." BioMed Research International 2020, no. 1 (2020): 9816142.
26. Jiang, Tao, Jian Ping Li, Amin Ul Haq, Abdus Saboor, and Amjad Ali. "A novel stacking approach for accurate detection of fake news." IEEE Access 9 (2021): 22626–22639.
27. Al-Yarimi, Fuad Ali Mohammed, Nabil Mohammed Ali Munassar, Mohammed Hasan Mohammed Bamashmos, and Mohammed Yousef Salem Ali. "Feature optimization by discrete weights for heart disease prediction using supervised learning." Soft Computing 25 (2021): 1821–1831.
28. Sarkar, Bikash Kanti. "Hybrid model for prediction of heart disease." Soft Computing 24 (2020): 1903–1925.
29. Miao, Kathleen H., Julia H. Miao, and George J. Miao. "Diagnosing coronary heart disease using ensemble machine learning." *International Journal of Advanced Computer Science and Applications* 7, no. 10 (2016).
30. Asuncion, Arthur, and David Newman. "UCI machine learning repository." (2007).
31. Ghauri, Sajjad Ahmed, Ijaz Mansoor Qureshi, and Aqdas Naveed Malik. "A novel approach for automatic modulation classification via hidden Markov models and Gabor features." Wireless Personal Communications 96 (2017): 4199–4216.

32. Sarfraz, Mubashar, Muhammad Farhan Sohail, Sheraz Alam, Muhammad Javvad ur Rehman, Sajjad Ahmed Ghauri, Khaled Rabie, Hasan Abbas, and Shuja Ansari. "Capacity optimization of next-generation UAV communication involving non-orthogonal multiple access." Drones 6, no. 9 (2022): 234.
33. Ghauri, Sajjad Ahmed. "Automatic modulation classification using feature based approach." PhD Dissertation, ISRA University Hyderabad, Islamabad Campus (2015).
34. Sohail, M., Sheraz Alam, Asad Hussain, Sajjad A. Ghauri, Mubashar Sarfraz, and M. Ahmed. "Multiuser detection: Comparative analysis of heuristic approach." International Journal of Advanced and Applied Scienes 4 (2017): 115–120.
35. Bilal, Ahmad, Shahzad Latif, Sajjad A. Ghauri, Oh-Young Song, Aaqif Afzaal Abbasi, and Tehmina Karamat. "Modified heuristic computational techniques for the resource optimization in cognitive radio networks (crns)." *Electronics* 12, no. 4 (2023): 973.
36. Zenodo. "Welfake dataset for fake news detection in text data." February 25, 2021.
37. Gravanis, Georgios, Athena Vakali, Konstantinos Diamantaras, and Panagiotis Karadais. "Behind the cues: A benchmarking study for fake news detection." Expert Systems with Applications 128 (2019): 201–213.
38. Buntain, Cody, and Jennifer Golbeck. "Automatically identifying fake news in popular twitter threads." In 2017 *IEEE International Conference on Smart Cloud (SmartCloud)*, pp. 208–215. IEEE, 2017.
39. Ahmed, Hadeer, Issa Traore, and Sherif Saad. "Detection of online fake news using n-gram analysis and machine learning techniques." In *Intelligent, Secure, and Dependable Systems in Distributed and Cloud Environments: First International Conference, ISDDC 2017,* Vancouver, BC, Canada, October 26–28, 2017, Proceedings 1, pp. 127–138. Springer International Publishing, 2017.
40. Khan, Inam Ullah, Ijaz Mansoor Qureshi, Muhammad Adnan Aziz, Tanweer Ahmad Cheema, and Syed Bilal Hussain Shah. "Smart IoT control-based nature inspired energy efficient routing protocol for flying ad hoc network (FANET)." IEEE Access 8 (2020): 56371–56378.
41. Arshi, Oroos, Akanksha Rai, Gauri Gupta, Jitendra Kumar Pandey, and Surajit Mondal. "IoT in energy: A comprehensive review of technologies, applications, and future directions." Peer-to-Peer Networking and Applications 1 (2024): 1–40.

3 An Intelligent Hybrid Blockchain Mechanism for IoT-Based Healthcare Applications in Blood Cancer Recurrence Detection

Mohsen Ghorbian and Saeid Ghorbian

3.1 INTRODUCTION

ALL is a type of blood cancer that occurs when the blood cells multiply irregularly and become unstable. The disease typically occurs in children and adolescents but can strike at any age due to the proliferation of malignant lymphocytes. ALL cancer is a rare disease but one of the most prevalent blood cancers in children. ALL cancer is much less common in adults, and only about 20% of ALL cancer cases occur in adults. However, the survival rates of adults with ALL cancer are generally lower than those of children. ALL cancer treatment can differ depending on the cancer's severity and the patient's characteristics. Many people with ALL cancer can recover and return to good health with the proper treatment [1]. IoT refers to a set of electronic devices connected to the Internet and capable of exchanging data with each other. These devices include sensors, medical devices, and other electronic devices. It is possible to utilize IoT to control and monitor cancer patients. Additionally, IoT can gather information regarding a patient's daily activities, such as sleep, activity, and food consumption, using sensors and wearable devices. Hence, using this information, physicians can gain a deeper understanding of the patient's condition and provide appropriate treatment or, if it is necessary, modify the treatment process. Cancer patients can benefit from IoT for improving control, monitoring, and treatment quality. Nevertheless, addressing data privacy and security issues and ensuring that sensitive patient data is protected from unauthorized access to utilize IoT effectively is essential [2]. ML is a subset of AI that enables computers to learn from and predict new data. They are used to diagnose and treat a wide range of diseases highly accurately. In cancer diagnosis, ML can identify patterns based on data collected from cancer patients that can assist in diagnosing cancer. In addition to diagnosis, ML can also be used to predict disease

DOI: 10.1201/9781003469896-3

recurrences. Hence, ML can use data collected from previous patients to identify patterns that help predict the likelihood of disease recurrence. As a result, doctors can better plan their treatment and follow-up of patients [3]. A blockchain is a digital-based technology that provides high levels of security and transparency for data exchange. Blockchain data is stored in blocks, each containing a list of transactions and a security code (hash) linked to previous blocks. As a result of its high level of security and transparency, this technology is widely used in healthcare applications. The blockchain can effectively maintain the security of sensitive patient data when controlling and monitoring patients via IoT. By storing patient data securely in interconnected blocks, blockchain identifies and tracks data changes or modifications. Hence, this will protect patients' privacy and prevent unauthorized access to their data. A blockchain-based system can also be applied to diagnose cancer and predict its recurrence using ML. Hence, patients' data can be securely stored in interconnected blocks using blockchain, and learning machines can be trained using this information. Therefore, this increases the accuracy and efficiency of the cancer diagnosis and the prediction of its recurrence. Consequently, blockchain technology can solve issues related to the privacy and security of sensitive patient data and concerns using IoT and ML [4]. This chapter attempts to provide an AI mechanism using IoT, ML, and blockchain technologies. With the presented AI mechanism, the challenges and concerns related to the use of new technologies in the field of health care are attempted to be addressed, including ensuring data security, protecting the identity of individuals, preventing unauthorized access to data, increasing the delay in checking the condition of patients by doctors, and uncertainty that patients can access doctors on time.

The structure of this chapter is as follows: As a starting point, the first part examines the necessary prerequisites such as cancer ALL, IoT, ML, and blockchain, and the features, capabilities, and capabilities of IoT, ML, and blockchain technology in the field of healthcare, especially in the diagnosis process of ALL cancer. The second part of this chapter describes ALL cancer, ML, blockchain, and IoT technologies in healthcare separately. The third part examines the application of blockchain and IoT in healthcare through subsets such as the overview of HLF blockchain technology, detection of ALL using various techniques, and classification approaches and techniques in ML. The fourth section comprehensively examines the incorporation of ML and IoT through blockchain. The fifth part of this chapter proposes an AI mechanism in IoT healthcare and describes it. As a final step, the sixth section concludes this explanation.

3.2 PRELIMINARIES

This section supplies information and terminology related to ALL Cancer and technologies like blockchain, ML, and the IoT. Additionally, these technologies have been discussed as solutions for detecting disease, monitoring and controlling affected patients, as well as protecting the privacy of individuals with acute lymphoblastic leukemia cancer, as well as demonstrating that the use of these technologies can increase the effectiveness of treatment and reduce the time required to identify recurrences.

3.2.1 ALL Cancer

ALL is a type of blood cancer that is more common in children and adolescents. In ALL, lymphoblastic cells (white blood cells) are abnormally produced and spread throughout the body. This disease mainly reduces the production of other types of blood cells, such as red blood cells, platelet cells, and other white blood cells, resulting in symptoms such as weakness and severe fatigue, chills, frequent infections, bleeding, and the risk of severe infections. Upon early detection of this disease, the patient can receive treatment sooner, and the chances of achieving a positive outcome are greater if treated promptly. By identifying the condition at an early stage, symptoms and complications of the disease may be reduced, and recurrence can be decreased likelihood. Treatment options for this cancer include chemotherapy, radiotherapy, and stem cell transplantation. These treatments are often combined. The duration of treatment varies from patient to patient and depends on the patient's age, gender, health status, and level of disease progression. Regarding the recurrence of this disease, it is essential to note that in some cases, cancer reappears due to remaining malignant cells in a patient's body. Upon completion of the initial treatment, patients must undergo post-treatment and preventative care and follow a strict medical follow-up order to prevent recurrence. ALL can be treated more effectively, and a patient's quality of life improves if detected early. Consequently, when persons experience suspicious symptoms, they should visit their doctor and obtain relevant tests, early diagnosis, and timely treatment. In addition to post-treatment care, follow-up tests, nutrition, regular physical activity, proper vaccination, and avoiding contact with chemicals known as risk factors are necessary to prevent ALL cancer from occurring. Generally, ALL is a severe disease that requires early diagnosis and effective treatment. Detecting and treating the disease promptly increases the probability of recovery and prevents recurrence. When persons encounter suspicious symptoms, the best thing to do is visit their doctor immediately and undergo the diagnosis and treatment procedures [5].

3.2.2 ML Technology

ML is a subset of AI that uses statistical and mathematical algorithms to teach machines to learn and make decisions based on the data and patterns they contain. ML allows machines to understand better the behavior and performance of various systems and processes and use this knowledge to make better decisions. ML technology can be helpful for the early diagnosis of various diseases in healthcare. This technology allows medical data to be analyzed automatically and rapidly, and patterns can be identified to aid in early diagnosis. By using ML, for instance, it is possible to analyze blood test results to identify patterns and predict the probability of a patient becoming ill based on them. The use of ML in the early diagnosis of diseases can have many benefits, including reducing diagnosis time, improving treatment results, reducing medical costs, and improving patients' quality of life. Using this technology for early disease diagnosis can increase the chance of recovery and reduce treatment time, resulting in a faster diagnosis process, a more effective treatment, and a more comfortable patient treatment experience. Many unique capabilities and features of ML have enhanced the use of this technology in the healthcare field. ML technology provides the following features in the process of diagnosing diseases:

- **More accuracy:** ML can diagnose diseases more accurately and precisely by analyzing patient data.
- **Use of large and complex data:** ML can identify patterns that can be used to diagnose diseases based on large and complex data sets.
- **Early diagnosis of the disease:** ML can assist in detecting diseases early, improving treatment, and reducing medical costs.
- **Ability to process data quickly:** ML can quickly and accurately make decisions based on that data.
- **Disease prediction:** ML can predict the probability of a disease occurrence in the future based on the patient's data.

As an advanced and powerful technology, ML can significantly improve the diagnosis and treatment of diseases and patients' quality of life. Hence, sufficient and accurate medical data must exist to utilize this technology effectively for the best results. A particular emphasis should also be placed on the privacy and security of medical data to ensure that these data can be used safely and in a manner that respects patients' rights [6].

3.2.3 Blockchain Technology

Blockchain technology is a technology for storing and managing data. Blockchain is a distributed system that stores data in blocks and links each block to the previous block. Hence, this ensures that the blockchain is protected from fraud and data changes and has high security. In general, blockchains can be divided into two types: public blockchains and permission-based blockchains. Public Blockchains are a distributed system capable of storing and verifying financial and non-financial transactions without needing a management center. In addition to reviewing, approving, or rejecting recorded transactions and data, anyone with access to such block chains can use them in e-commerce, supply chains, internet payments, etc. Bitcoin is one of the most widely known public blockchains. Bitcoin uses blockchain technology, and all transactions are recorded and verified publicly without needing a management center. Another type of public blockchain is Ethereum, a platform used to create and manage applications that run on the blockchain. Solidity is the programming language for developing Ethereum smart contracts and applications. Generally, public blockchains are used in many fields due to their high levels of security, transparency, and lack of management centers. Due to their lack of dependence on companies and organizations, these blockchains are considered a new method of creating trust and transparency in the digital world [7]. A permission-based blockchain is another type generally designed to be suitable for use in organizations and businesses. The right to access the blockchain and verify transactions in this type of blockchain is granted to a limited number of individuals, often including the organization's members. Users need access permissions from blockchain management to enter these types of blockchains. HLF is one of the most prominent permission-based blockchains, developed by the Linux Foundation (Linux Foundation) and designed for use in organizations and corporations. As a development platform, HLF allows applications using various languages like Go, Java, and Node.js to run on the blockchain. This blockchain has the characteristics of transparency, security, reliability, and repeatability. Permission-based blockchains are more secure than public blockchains because they are authenticated only to those with access. Also, these types of blockchains are usually used for specific applications such as supply chains, insurance, banking, etc. A permission-based blockchain is typically used in organizations and companies because it provides higher security and greater control over access to data. Blockchain can serve many purposes in healthcare and cancer diagnosis as a new technology. One application of blockchain in this field is to store and share the medical data of cancer patients. Many different systems contain the medical data of patients, and many of these systems are not coordinated with each other, causing difficulties in the diagnosis and treatment of patients. Patient's medical data can be stored in a distributed and integrated system using blockchain. Hence, doctors and health professionals can effectively diagnose and treat diseases by providing full access to patients' medical data. It is also possible to utilize blockchain technology to conduct research in the field of cancer diagnosis and treatment. Data can be stored and shared automatically without the need for intermediaries, and these data can contribute to the field of cancer diagnosis and treatment [8].

3.2.4 IoT Technology

In the IoT, devices, and sensors are connected to the Internet via wireless and Internet technologies to send and receive data automatically without human intervention. By using wireless and Internet technologies, these devices can communicate with one another and the communication network and exchange data. The IoT has three main components: devices, the network, and the cloud. IoT devices include sensors, wearables, wireless devices, door openers, home appliances, etc. These devices can automatically transmit useful data to the Internet. The IoT network includes devices that can receive data sent from different devices and receive and store this data in the cloud platform with the help of communication protocols such as MQTT and HTTP [9]. The IoT cloud platform includes services that assist the IoT in collecting and analyzing data and automatically transferring it to machines using ML algorithms and AI mechanisms. Due to its wide range of applications in many industries, the IoT is an effective technology in healthcare and cancer diagnosis. The following are some instances of the types of IoT and their applications in the fields of healthcare and cancer diagnosis:

- **Types of IoT:**
  - **Medical devices:** These include sensors for measuring blood pressure, blood sugar, heart rate, etc.
  - **Wearable devices:** These include smart watches, smart bands, etc.
  - **Smart city devices:** include innovative composters, intelligent street lights, etc.
  - **Household devices:** These include intelligent refrigerators, door openers, etc.

- **Applications of IoT in the field of healthcare:**
  - **Patient health monitoring:** Medical and wearable devices can monitor patients' health and automatically alert physicians.
  - **Improving the performance of hospitals:** Smart city devices can be utilized to improve the performance of hospitals and provide better facilities for patients and health care professionals.
  - **Monitoring and controlling environmental conditions:** Through household devices and smart cities, it is possible to monitor environmental conditions, determine optimal health conditions, and prevent the spreading of diseases.
- **Applications of IoT in cancer diagnosis:**
  - **Health monitoring:** Wearable devices can monitor a person's health and detect diseases early. For instance, using heart rate monitors, adverse symptoms can be detected and helpful in detecting cancer at an early stage.
  - **Medical imaging:** Using medical devices such as intelligent imaging machines, high-quality X-ray images can be taken from patients, and cancer can be detected using intelligent algorithms.
  - **Treatment monitoring:** Wearable devices and smart sensors can help monitor a person's treatment and be used for better diagnosis and treatment.

Generally, the IoT is a new technology with many potential applications in the medical field, particularly in cancer diagnosis. It is possible to improve the performance of hospitals, monitor and control environmental conditions, and diagnose cancer using this technology [10].

3.3 BLOCKCHAIN AND IoT IN HEALTHCARE

Combining blockchain and IoT technologies by collecting patients' medical data from IoT wearable devices and storing them in blockchain can significantly improve healthcare quality. Combining blockchain and IoT technologies by collecting patients' medical data from IoT wearable devices and storing them in blockchain can significantly improve healthcare quality. In other words, embedded sensors on IoT wearable devices can automatically monitor and collect patients' health data stored on a blockchain database. Therefore, it is possible to use blockchain technology to provide secure access to medical data collected by IoT devices and share this data with authenticated individuals like doctors, patients, and hospitals. Permission-based blockchain technology, such as HLF, increases trust in sharing data in the healthcare field. For instance, Blockchain can allow doctors to ensure that patient data is accurate and reliable and treat patients more effectively. By combining blockchain and IoT technologies, it is also possible to verify the validity of the sent data and provide assurance in the accuracy of data collected by wearable devices and health monitoring sensors of patients. Hence, with trust in data, doctors can improve their state of patient's health in the best way [11]. IoT and blockchain technologies can be used in healthcare in two different ways: first, as a centralized medical data system, and second, as a distributed medical data system. The centralized medical data system stores all medical data regarding patients in a centralized location. It allows verified people, such as doctors, patients, and hospitals, to access this data through the blockchain [12]. With access to all of the patient's medical data in one place, doctors can make the best decisions regarding their patients' treatment. A distributed medical data system in which patients' medical data is stored on multiple blockchains and connected via IoT networks. Doctors can access patients' medical data across a network using this system and make the best decisions regarding their care. Finally, combining IoT and blockchain in healthcare can improve the quality of medical services, increase the security of medical data, and reduce the cost of treatment by improving the quality of medical services [13].

3.3.1 Overview of HLF Blockchain Technology

The HLF permission-based blockchain is one of the open-source blockchain technologies supported by the Linux Foundation. It is recognized as one of the most influential blockchain tools for business use. It was developed to address the concerns of traditional blockchains, such as the necessity of centralizing the network and connecting it to a super blockchain, which can lead to a lack of security, reduced speed, and unreliability issues. Using permission-based blockchains such as HLF technology solves these problems. Permission-based blockchains ensure network security and prevent unauthorized access by requiring all network participants to have permission to access the network. The HLF structure utilizes a private channel architecture. As a result, network participants can communicate privately, and only the data shared between them will be stored in the blockchain. Hence, this can prevent the problem of excess data volume associated with traditional blockchains. It is also important to note that HLF supports Sidechain. In this system, instead of all data being stored in a single blockchain, the data related to each participant is stored in a little blockchain. Hence, this can avoid slow data mining issues in traditional blockchains. HLF can be a secure, reliable, and scalable blockchain technology in many markets and industries [14]. This technology can be an excellent choice for businesses seeking trustworthy blockchain solutions. HLF has several unique characteristics that distinguish it from other blockchain protocols, including:

- **Privacy:** HLF uses a privacy and security system to ensure the privacy and security of its network. It allows network participants to access the data for which they are authorized to do so.
- **Flexibility:** HLF assists companies in establishing and managing their blockchain applications and improving efficiency and security across industries. Furthermore, this technology supports a network and member management system that can be tailored to meet the needs of companies.
- **High speed:** HLF allows companies to process more transactions per second than they can using traditional blockchain technologies.
- **Smart contract support:** HLF supports Smart Contracts, enabling companies to create and manage their applications. This technology also supports multiple programming languages, enabling companies to choose the language for their applications.
- **High security:** The HLF technology utilizes strong encryption algorithms to protect network data, access management, and authentication mechanisms.

- **Adaptability:** The HLF allows companies to customize, update, and modify their blockchain applications to their requirements easily.
- **Flexibility in data management:** HLF companies can manage their data according to their needs and store data on the blockchain flexibly and effectively. Also, this protocol provides data management tools that allow companies to quickly and efficiently manage their data on the blockchain.

Components in HLF assist in managing and simplifying blockchain networks in implementation. It allows companies to write code for different parts, such as smart contracts, in separate files and then combine them. Companies and organizations can use components to keep the various components of the contract in separate files. As a result, their code becomes simpler, more readable, and easier to manage when they use HLF tools to combine these components and create their smart contract as a whole. Also, using components in HLF allows companies and organizations to rewrite the code related to different parts of the contract without affecting other parts. Doing so allows them to easily update any part of the contract that needs to be changed without affecting the other parts [15]. Figure 3.1 illustrates the architecture of HLF, which identifies the main components of the framework.

- **Ordering Service**:

  The Orderer Service manages the production order and verification of blockchain blocks. The Orderer Service creates a new block by verifying

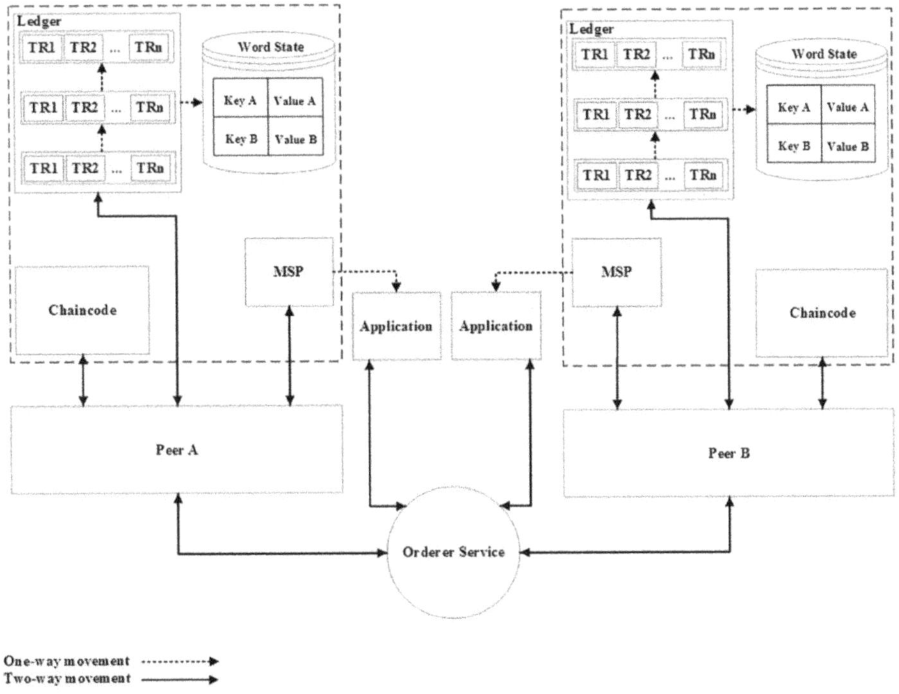

FIGURE 3.1 The critical components in the HLF architecture.

transactions created by network users and sending them to the Orderer Service. After receiving the order, the Orderer Service creates the relevant block and transmits it to every network node so it can be stored in its blockchain. The Orderer Service consists of two main parts:

- **Consensus layer**: In this layer, decisions are made regarding generating and verifying blockchain blocks. It is responsible for validating the order in which blockchain blocks are created. As part of the Consensus Layer, HLF uses the Kafka or solo Algorithm to ensure that all blocks are verified in order across all paths within the network and are ready for use in the following.
- **Delivery layer**: In this layer, the blocks confirmed in the Consensus Layer are sent to all network nodes to be stored in their blockchains [16].

- **Ordering Service:**

  Peers are one of the most critical components of the HLF blockchain network. They execute smart contract transactions, receive verified blocks, and add them to their blockchains. There are several roles that Peers play to accomplish this:

  - **Anchor Peer**: Each blockchain network has an Anchor Peer that communicates with Anchor Peers of other blockchain networks to share information. Anchor Peers play an essential role in communication between different blockchain networks.
  - **Validator Peer**: In the HLF blockchain network, Validator Peers are responsible for verifying new blocks. After receiving new blocks, they verify that the blocks are valid, and when the blocks are correct, they add them to their blockchain.
  - **Gossip Peer**: In the HLF blockchain network, gossip peers exchange information between Peers. By doing so, all Peers in the network are kept informed and have access to the latest information.
  - **Endorser Peer**: The Endorser Peers are responsible for executing smart contracts. Before creating a transaction, the transaction is sent to the Endorser Peers for the execution of the corresponding smart contract and the return of the result to the transaction for confirmation [17].

- **Ledger:**

  Ledgers in HLF are responsible for storing and managing blockchain data. Each blockchain in HLF includes a ledger that permanently stores all transactions. The Ledger component of HLF utilizes two types of databases. The Ledger component of HLF utilizes two databases, State and Transaction databases. The State Database in HLF stores data generated by smart contract transactions. The database stores these data in key-value format. Each data contains a state key and a value corresponding to the state key. When a smart contract creates a transaction, the state database is updated. The Transaction Database in HLF stores the details of transactions created in the blockchain network. Among the information contained within this database are the transaction ID, the time at which the transaction was created, the name of the relevant smart contract, and the parameters sent to it. As a result, the Transaction Database serves as a log for all transactions executed on the blockchain system [18].

- **Membership Service Provider (MSP):**
  MSP is a service provider that manages and authenticates its network's members. HLF provides a unique identity for every member of the blockchain network, which determines their permissions and accesses to execute transactions and access network data. In HLF, the MSP is responsible for the following tasks:
  - **Access management**: MSP's access management system utilizes Membership and Role-Based Access Control (RBAC). These tools allow access to be determined by the role and permissions of each network member.
  - **Management of certificates**: The MSP uses digital certificates to authenticate network members. These certificates are issued by the CA (Certificate Authority) service in HLF and are managed by the MSP as a service provider [19].
- **Chaincode**:
  Chaincode or Smart Contracts in HLF is a central component of the blockchain network that facilitates the definition and execution of smart contracts. Chaincode is divided into two types System and Application Chaincode in HLF. System Chaincode in HLF manages the blockchain network and performs basic operations such as adding and removing network members, creating channels, executing main transactions, and managing access to various network components. Application Chaincode functions as a basis for defining smart contracts in HLF. Smart contracts can specify a data structure, access rules, and operations that can be performed based on the network's requirements [20].

3.3.2 Detection of ALL Using Various Techniques

Blood cancers such as ALL are caused by gene changes that promote blood cell division and growth. Children and teenagers are more likely to experience this type of cancer, which has symptoms such as fatigue, hard breathing, and swelling in the neck, digestive system, and body for at least one month. Several methods are used for treating ALL cancer, including chemotherapy, radiotherapy, bone marrow cell transplantation (BMT), and new and innovative drugs. Chemotherapy involves prescribing drugs to patients that inhibit cancer cell growth. In radiotherapy, high-energy rays destroy cancer cells as well. In a myeloid cell transplant, healthy myeloid cells are transferred from a healthy individual to the patient so that healthy blood cells can grow instead of cancerous cells [21]. In addition, new and innovative drugs are also available to treat ALL types of cancer. This disease can be diagnosed using a variety of methods, including:

- **Blood test:** ALL cancer is diagnosed through a blood test. This test measures the level of white blood cells, the level of platelets, and the level of hemoglobin in the blood. High levels of white blood cells and low levels of hemoglobin indicate the presence of ALL cancer.

- **Bone marrow test:** In this method, a small sample of bone marrow is taken, and then the cancer cells are examined under a microscope. This test is one of the most important for diagnosing ALL cancer.
- **Biopsy:** A biopsy removes a sample of suspicious tissue or cells for analysis in a laboratory. A bone marrow biopsy is generally used to diagnose ALL cancer.
- **Imaging:** In some cases, imaging may also be used to diagnose ALL cancers, including radiography, computed tomography (CT), magnetic resonance imaging (MRI), and positron emission tomography (PET).

Several factors may influence the development of ALL cancer, making prevention of this type of cancer a complex issue. ALL cancer can be prevented by leading a healthy life and following a healthy diet, consulting with your doctor, and taking preventive tests if necessary. Furthermore, occupational health and safety, avoiding exposure to hazardous chemicals or radiation, and preventing viral infections can all effectively prevent the development of this type of cancer [22].

3.3.3 Classification Approaches and Techniques in ML

By using ML technology, laws, and patterns can be discovered that can be used to predict new data. ML can accomplish this task with various algorithms based on existing approaches that obtained results vary according to the data type and the desired problem to be variable. Therefore, the selection type of approach for implementation by ML must be based on considered goals. Following is an examination of the approaches used in the ML technology.

- **Unsupervised learning**: In unsupervised learning, learning algorithms attempt to discover the patterns in the data automatically and without the need for labels or training examples, according to the input data. Generally, unsupervised algorithms can identify and predict new examples without any instructions. In AI, unsupervised learning is one of the methods used in various applications, such as natural language processing, big data analysis, imaging, and pattern recognition. There are several famous algorithms in unsupervised learning, including K-Means Clustering, Density-Based Spatial Clustering of Applications with Noise (DBSCAN), Principal Component Analysis (PCA), Independent Component Analysis (ICA), Autoencoders Non-negative Matrix Factorization (NMF), Latent Dirichlet Allocation (LDA), K-Nearest Neighbors (KNN), and Expectation-Maximization (EM) [23].
- **Reinforcement learning**: The reinforcement learning agent interacts automatically with the environment without input data or labels to learn the appropriate behavior to obtain a reward based on the environment. In reinforcement learning, the agent receives a reward for performing a particular action and attempts to learn the appropriate behavior to obtain further rewards. AI uses reinforcement learning in various applications, including

computer games, robotics, flight control, resource management, and network management. There are several main algorithms in reinforcement learning, including Proximal Policy Optimization (PPO), Trust Region Policy Optimization (TRPO), Asynchronous Advantage Actor-Critic (A3C), Deterministic Policy Gradient (DPG), Upper Confidence Bound (UCB), and Thompson Sampling [24].

- **Supervised learning**: In supervised learning, learning algorithms learn the relationships between inputs and outputs using input data with a label or correct answer. In other words, in supervised learning, labels related to input data are provided as training examples for learning algorithms. AI uses supervised learning processes to accomplish various tasks, including pattern recognition, language processing, and facial recognition. There are several prominent algorithms in supervised learning, including Linear Regression, Logistic Regression, Decision Tree, Random Forest, Naive Bayes, Support Vector Machines (SVM), Gradient Boosting Machines (GBMs), Extreme Gradient Boosting (XGBoost), AdaBoost, Gradient Descent, and Stochastic Gradient Descent (SGD) [25].
- **Neural networks**: In ML, neural networks are one of the most commonly used methods, which are based on the structure and function of the human nervous system. Essentially, neural networks are mathematical models consisting of layers of neurons that, using learning algorithms, can identify hidden patterns in data based on input data. Among the many applications of neural networks in image processing, they are used to process natural language, pattern recognition and prediction, speech processing, computer games, and many other tasks. There are several primary algorithms in neural networks, including Perceptron, Multilayer Perceptron (MLP), Convolutional Neural Networks (CNNs), Recurrent Neural Networks (RNNs), Long Short-Term Memory (LSTM), Gated Recurrent Unit (GRU), Autoencoders Generative Adversarial Networks (GANs), and Deep Belief Networks (DBNs) [26].

3.4 INCORPORATING ML AND IoT THROUGH BLOCKCHAIN

Incorporating ML and IoT through blockchain is one of the most critical issues in healthcare technology due to its high potential to maintain data security, transparency, reliability, and accuracy. Due to the strong connection between blockchain and concepts such as security, transparency, and trust, researchers can easily use this data to train and improve ML algorithms based on the data collected by IoT devices recorded in blocks of the blockchain network. As part of incorporating ML and IoT through blockchain, data collected by IoT devices are chained and recorded in blockchain blocks. Each block contains information from collected data that can be analyzed using ML algorithms. In this way, new patterns can be detected in collected data using these algorithms, and future behaviors can be predicted. Consequently, by combining these technologies, researchers can train ML algorithms with more accurate data and predict future behaviors more accurately. Utilizing blockchain as a data storage technology enables researchers to benefit from high security in data storage and prevent unlicensed access and change data in IoT systems by ensuring that all previous blocks must be changed to change existing data on one block. Furthermore, blockchain allows researchers to utilize the data collected by IoT devices without the need to trust other devices, and it dramatically solves the concerns of data and information shared being misused by patients and medical centers. Managing the large amount of data collected by IoT devices is one of the main challenges in Incorporating ML and IoT through blockchain. Therefore, it is possible to overcome this challenge using data compression algorithms. Furthermore, because the calculation of ML algorithms involves a large amount of processing and calculations, IoT devices will need powerful processors to be capable of running the algorithms. Aside from the benefits of Incorporating ML with IoT through blockchain, there are challenges. For instance, blockchain requires powerful processing to support a large number of IoT devices at the same time. Hence, the collected data must also be transmitted to the blockchain servers promptly and uninterruptedly with high bandwidth over high-speed communication networks [27]. Incorporating ML and IoT through blockchain can also provide a solution for rapidly diagnosing patients with ALL cancer. Thus, the combined use of these technologies and their features can be used as proposed mechanisms for addressing the challenges and problems associated with maintaining, caring for, controlling, and monitoring patients' health in the post-recovery period.

3.5 AI MECHANISM IN IoT HEALTHCARE

In the relapse of ALL cancer, adult lymphocyte cells normally produced in the bone marrow multiply inappropriately and increase the number of healthy cells in the bloodstream. The body produces some proteins naturally, which may be used as indicators of disease diagnosis and follow-up in some cases. In cured ALL cancer patients where cancer recurrence occurs, C-reactive protein (CRP) is one of the proteins that are produced in an increased amount in their blood. As a marker of inflammation in the body, this protein can be used to diagnose and follow up inflammatory and infectious diseases. Some studies have shown that the level of CRP in the blood of ALL patients with relapse is higher. Several factors contribute to the recurrence of ALL cancer, and other tests must be conducted to diagnose and follow up on the condition; however, CRP can be considered an essential indicator of ALL cancer recurrence. CRP is a plasma glycoprotein produced in response to inflammation and infections caused by bacteria, viruses, and parasites. A higher level of this protein is found in the blood in cases of inflammation such as rheumatoid arthritis, atherosclerosis, cancer, and bacterial and viral infections caused by the liver. According to some studies, patients with relapse have a higher level of CRP in their blood, so the high CRP level can be used as a diagnostic indicator of ALL recurrence. The normal level of CRP in healthy people's blood is less than 10 mg/L. However, a CRP value higher than 100 mg/L in the blood can be considered a marker of ALL cancer recurrence [28]. This chapter has attempted to propose a mechanism for early detection of ALL cancer recurrence by utilizing IoT, Blockchain, and ML technologies. The proposed artificial intelligence (AI) mechanism measures CRP levels in patient blood by taking blood from the patient multiple times at different intervals. Next, the proposed intelligent mechanism attempts to implement ML techniques on the patient data received. By implementing ML techniques on the data received from the patient, the proposed AI mechanism can predict the situation and the trend of increasing the CRP value in the time intervals when the data is received. The proposed AI mechanism can potentially be used by several users simultaneously. Hence, the proposed AI mechanism receives the results of implementing ML techniques to prioritize patients' access to physicians. In other words, it receives the prediction of the increase in CRP levels in their blood. The patient's condition in the proposed AI mechanism is divided into four states: acute above 100 mg/L, becoming acute between 50 and 100 mg/L, needing further investigation between 10 and 50 mg/L, and normally less than 10 mg/L. Thus, it tries to prioritize patients obtaining access to doctors based on the determined states and the predictions he has received based on the patient's condition. The access process is based on prioritization, so the patients for whom the predicted process is acute are highly prioritized. Then, the following priorities are in the order of the states towards becoming acute, requiring further investigation and normal examinations. In this regard, the proposed AI mechanism aims to reduce the time it takes patients with an acute diagnosis to access physicians. Therefore, with this AI mechanism, it will be possible to reduce the delays caused by the access of people with bad conditions to physicians, which can result in a faster start of the treatment process and ultimately increase the effectiveness. Consequently, the proposed AI mechanism and the stated advantages can significantly solve the problems caused by the lack of physicians and specialists in utilizing new technologies such as the IoT to solve these issues. A detailed analysis of the implementation steps of the AI mechanism proposed in Figure 3.2 will be presented below. Figure 3.3 illustrates the proposed mechanism architecture.

In the proposed AI mechanism, patients would receive their blood samples using IoT devices that are capable of measuring CRP (step 1). IoT devices can connect to a system with a blockchain network. Therefore, they send a request to connect to the network. In the network, a mechanism is considered in which users must first be authenticated by the authentication mechanism before accessing the network, ensuring only authorized IoT devices can access the network (step 2). After checking and confirming the identity of the IoT devices via an authentication mechanism, a response is generated informing the applicant that the device has been approved (step 3). Next, to access the blockchain network, IoT devices act as an application. After the Endorser nodes approve IoT device requests, they can request to insert their information into the Orderer Service. Requests are queued and executed in order as part of the Orderer Service (step 4). After placing the requests in the queue, the Orderer Services sends the available requests to Chaincode for execution, and this process is communicated through a request (step 5). When Chaincode receives a request from the Orderer Service, it attempts to provide the conditions for implementing the request as a query and sends it to the ledger (step 6). Upon receiving the request to insert information in the form of a query, Ledger attempts to store the data, and once the data storage process is successful, it sends a message in the form of a response to Chaincode (step 7). After receiving a response from the Ledger

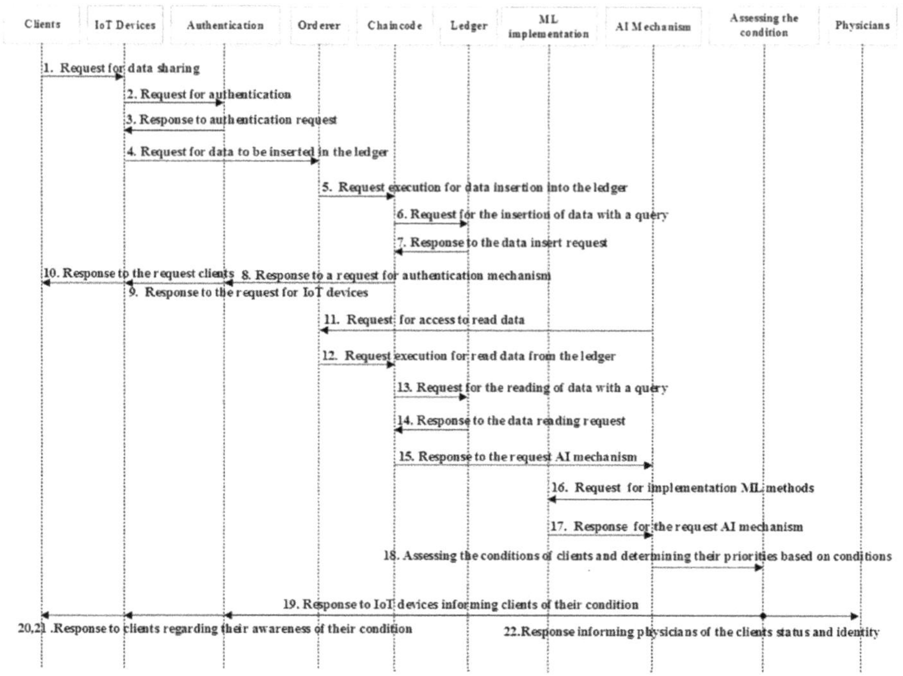

FIGURE 3.2 AI mechanism for patient data sharing with ML, HLF, and IoT healthcare.

that the data has been successfully inserted, Chaincode creates a message in the form of a response and sends it to the Authentication mechanism (step 8). As soon as the authentication mechanism receives a response, it attempts to send a message to the IoT devices (step 9). Upon receiving the message, IoT devices display a response to inform users that the process of storing their data has been completed (step 10). The proposed AI mechanism can be utilized simultaneously by several users. Consequently, once users enter information about their CRP level, the artificial intelligence mechanism first attempts to read the blockchain data to determine which patients with bad condition health have the priority of access to doctors. As a result, it attempts to request the data from the Orderer Service (step 11). The Orderer Service attempts to create a request for Chaincode after receiving a request for data from the AI mechanism (step 12). To respond to the request, Chaincode creates a Query and asks the Ledger to read the requested data (step 13). Upon receiving the request and reading the data, Ledger attempts to inform Chaincode of the readiness of the desired data by creating a response (step 14). As soon as Chaincode receives a response to its request, it attempts to inform the AI mechanism that the requested data is available by creating a response (step 15). As soon as the AI mechanism receives the desired data, it uses ML techniques to predict the trend in CRP increase in patients by analyzing data. Thus, by sending a request, the desired data is sent to the implementation ML mechanism (step 16). ML techniques are implemented in this step on the desired data and information of

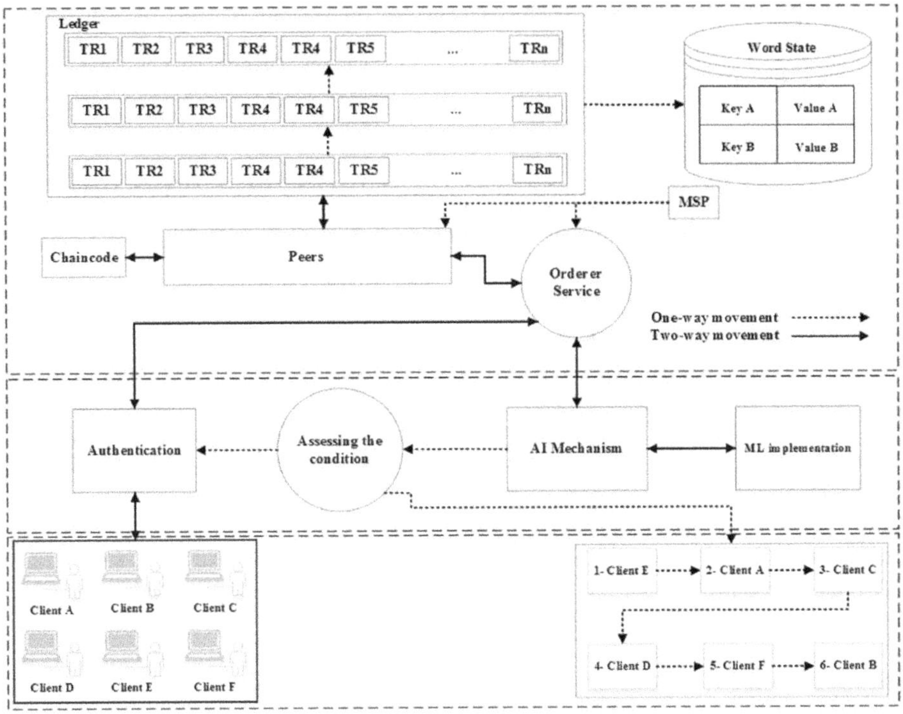

FIGURE 3.3 AI mechanism architecture for sharing patient data with HLF, ML, and IoT healthcare.

the AI mechanism to predict the trend of increasing CRP levels in patients and then send the resulting results as a response to the AI mechanism (step 17). Upon receiving the results, the AI mechanism requests that the assessing condition mechanism determine the patient's condition (step 18). At this step, their condition is evaluated and prioritized based on the prediction of the increasing trend of CRP in their blood. Therefore, patients with a CRP level greater than 100 mg/L will receive a higher priority for accessing physicians. By determining the priorities, they attempt to inform patients with a higher priority about their condition. Therefore, a request is sent to the authentication mechanism (step 19). Next, to inform the patients about their condition and the need to contact the physicians immediately, a request is sent to the IoT devices, and then the IoT devices inform the patients about their condition by showing a warning message (steps 20 and 21). Lastly, a message is sent from the assessing condition mechanism to the doctors, which specifies the priority of the patients, and the physicians will communicate with the patients by the priority determined (step 22).

In this manner, patients with acute conditions will have the right and priority to access doctors sooner using the AI mechanism. However, delaying access to doctors will not be as effective for patients with other conditions as it is for acutely ill patients. By enabling patients to access doctors more quickly, they will be able to begin their treatment process more quickly and with less delay, which in turn will increase their chances of surviving and preventing disease recurrence.

3.6 CONCLUSION

Since healthcare directly relates to human health, it is always considered a sensitive field. In this regard, there are always challenges and concerns arising from hospitals' lack of equipment and medical staff. When a person suffers from a severe disease such as cancer, they must be under constant supervision and care following the completion of the treatment period. A type of cancer known as ALL is most prevalent in children. It is important for people who become ill with this disease to be monitored and controlled by a physician if they recover from it since the disease can recur. In light of the healthcare shortages and concerns and the large number of patients present, doctors and medical centers can only control and monitor some of them. Any delay in diagnosis can result in irreparable costs for patients who may experience disease recurrence. Hence, emerging technologies are always considered a solution to reduce existing challenges and concerns. As part of the solution, doc-tors, by using IoT technology, can control and monitor patients remotely, and by using ML can predict disease recurrence and early detection. In this chapter, an at-tempt has been made to present an AI mechanism using new technologies such as the IoT, ML, and blockchain. This mechanism aims to address to the greatest extent possible the challenges and concerns that exist in the medical field for patients. The proposed artificial intelligence mechanism allows people to communicate with doctors and medical centers remotely and to share their health information. This proposed AI mechanism has attempted to secure shared data and protect patient's identity and privacy. All patient information is stored on the blockchain, and the data protection process is carried out through permission-based blockchains such as HLF. A proposed AI mechanism examines the data patients have stored on the blockchain and uses ML to determine the risk of ALL cancer recurrence by checking the level of CRP in their blood. By examining the results obtained from applying ML technology, the proposed AI mechanism attempts to categorize the condition of patients. Hence, this enables the patient's condition to be divided into four states such as acute, becoming acute, requiring further investigation, and normal. As a result, by prioritizing the condition of patients, the proposed AI mechanism attempts to give the highest priority to patients diagnosed with acute conditions. Accordingly, based on the considered communication mechanism, patients with higher priority will be selected as those who can access doctors and specialists more quickly and without delay. Those whose disease recurrence is severe and acute will be able to communicate with their doctor immediately and under their physician's direct supervision and control as part of this proposal.

In the future, using cloud computing technology to increase accessibility for a wider audience will be the basis of the proposed approach. Also, in attention to simplifying the implementation process and considering approaches that can significantly reduce the amount of energy consumed by IoT devices, the availability time of these devices can increase.

REFERENCES

1. Chiu, M., Taurino, G., Bianchi, M. G., Kilberg, M. S., & Bussolati, O. Asparagine synthetase in cancer: Beyond acute lymphoblastic leukemia. *Frontiers in Oncology* (2020). https://doi.org/10.3389/fonc.2019.01480
2. Selvaraj, S., & Sundaravaradhan, S. Challenges and opportunities in IoT healthcare systems: A systematic review. *SN Applied Sciences* 2, no. 1 (2020): 139.
3. Char, D. S., Abràmoff, M. D., & Feudtner, C. Identifying ethical considerations for machine learning healthcare applications. *The American Journal of Bioethics* (2020).
4. Waheed, N., He, X., Ikram, M., Usman, M., Hashmi, S. S., & Usman, M. Security and privacy in IoT using machine learning and blockchain: Threats and countermeasures. *ACM Computing Surveys (CSUR)* (2020).
5. Coccaro, N., Anelli, L., Zagaria, A., Specchia, G., & Albano, F. Next-generation sequencing in acute lymphoblastic leukemia. *International Journal of Molecular Sciences* (2019).
6. Callahan, A., & Shah, N. H. (2017). Machine learning in healthcare. In *Key Advances in Clinical Informatics* (pp. 279–291). Academic Press (2017).
7. Vujičić, D., Jagodić, D., & Ranđić, S. Blockchain technology, bitcoin, and Ethereum: A brief overview. In *2018 17th International Symposium Infoteh-Jahorina (Infoteh)*, East Sarajevo (pp. 1–6). IEEE (2018).
8. Kaur, J., Rani, R., & Kalra, N. Blockchain-based framework for secured storage, sharing, and querying of electronic healthcare records. *Concurrency and Computation: Practice and Experience* (2021).
9. Sarierao, B. S., & Prakasarao, A. Smart healthcare monitoring system using MQTT protocol. In *2018 3rd International Conference for Convergence in Technology (I2CT)*, Pune, India (pp. 1–5). IEEE (2018).
10. Onasanya, A., & Elshakankiri, M. Smart integrated IoT healthcare system for cancer care. *Wireless Networks* (2021).
11. Ghorbian, M., & Ghobaei-Arani, M. A. Blockchain-enabled serverless approach for IoT healthcare applications. In Nour El Madhoun, Ioanna Dionysiou, Emmanuel Bertin (eds). *Serverless Computing: Principles and Paradigms* (pp. 193–218). Cham: Springer International Publishing (2023).
12. Vyas, S., Shabaz, M., Pandit, P., Parvathy, L. R., & Ofori, I. Integration of Artificial Intelligence and blockchain technology in healthcare and agriculture. *Journal of Food Quality* (2022).
13. Celesti, A., Ruggeri, A., Fazio, M., Galletta, A., Villari, M., & Romano, A. Blockchain-based healthcare workflow for tele-medical laboratory in federated hospital IoT clouds. *Sensors* (2020).
14. Patsonakis, C., Terzi, S., Moschos, I., Ioannidis, D., Votis, K., & Tzovaras, D. Permissioned blockchains and virtual nodes for reinforcing trust between aggregators and prosumers in energy demand response scenarios. In *2019 IEEE International Conference on Environment and Electrical Engineering and 2019 IEEE Industrial and Commercial Power Systems Europe (EEEIC/I&CPS Europe)*, Genova, Italy (pp. 1–6). IEEE (2019).
15. Honar Pajooh, H., Rashid, M., Alam, F., & Demidenko, S. Multi-layer blockchain-based security architecture for internet of things. *Sensors* (2021).
16. Foschini, L., Gavagna, A., Martuscelli, G., & Montanari, R. Hyperledger fabric block-chain: Chaincode performance analysis. In *ICC 2020-2020 IEEE International Conference on Communications (ICC)*, Dublin, Ireland (pp. 1–6). IEEE (2020).
17. Zulkifl, Z., Khan, F., Tahir, S., Afzal, M., Iqbal, W., Rehman, A., & Almuhaideb, A. M. FBASHI: Fuzzy and blockchain-based adaptive security for healthcare IoTs. *IEEE Access* (2022).

18. Palm, E., Schelén, O., & Bodin, U. Selective blockchain transaction pruning and state derivability. In *2018 Crypto Valley Conference on Blockchain Technology (CVCBT)* (pp. 31–40). IEEE (2018).
19. Uddin, M., Salah, K., Jayaraman, R., Pesic, S., & Ellahham, S. Blockchain for drug traceability: Architectures and open challenges. *Health Informatics Journal* (2021).
20. Ghorbian, M., & Ghobaei-Arani, M. A blockchain-enabled serverless security mechanism for IoT-based drones. In Nour El Madhoun, Ioanna Dionysiou, Emmanuel Bertin (eds). *Building Cybersecurity Applications with Blockchain and Smart Contracts* (pp. 55–82). Cham: Springer Nature Switzerland (2024).
21. Hamdi, M., Wen, S., & Yang, Y. BTM: Boundary Trimming Module for temporal action detection. *Electronics* (2022).
22. Lauri, C., Tamminga, M., Glaudemans, A. W., Juárez Orozco, L. E., Erba, P. A., Jutte, P. C., Lipsky, B. A., IJzerman, M. J., Signore, A., & Slart, R. H. Detection of osteomyelitis in the diabetic foot by imaging techniques: A systematic review and meta-analysis comparing MRI, white blood cell scintigraphy, and FDG-PET. *Diabetes Care* (2017).
23. Arafa, A., El-Fishawy, N., Badawy, M., & Radad, M. RN-Autoencoder: Reduced Noise Autoencoder for classifying imbalanced cancer genomic data. *Journal of Biological Engineering* (2023).
24. Zeng, Y., Cai, R., Sun, F., Huang, L., & Hao, Z. A survey on causal reinforcement learning. arXiv preprint arXiv:2302.05209 (2023).
25. Jaiswal, A., Babu, A. R., Zadeh, M. Z., Banerjee, D., & Makedon, F. A survey on contrastive self-supervised learning. *Technologies* (2020).
26. Li, Z., Liu, F., Yang, W., Peng, S., & Zhou, J. A survey of convolutional neural networks: Analysis, applications, and prospects. *IEEE Transactions on Neural Networks and Learning Systems* (2021).
27. Jamshidi, M. B., Ebadpour, M., & Moghani, M. M. Cancer digital twins in metaverse. In *2022 20th International Conference on Mechatronics-Mechatronika (ME)* (pp. 1–6). IEEE (2022).
28. Dolan, R. D., McSorley, S. T., Horgan, P. G., Laird, B., & McMillan, D. C. The role of the systemic inflammatory response in predicting outcomes in patients with advanced inoperable cancer: Systematic review and meta-analysis. *Critical Reviews in Oncology/Hematology* (2017).

4 Comprehensive Solution for the Management of Chronic Kidney Disease

Application of IoT-Assisted Technology

Shikha and U.V. Kiran

4.1 INTRODUCTION

Chronic kidney disease (CKD) is a persistent condition characterized by a gradual loss of renal function, leading to the buildup of fluid and waste products in the body (Romagnani et al., 2017). This condition affects millions of people worldwide and is a major public health issue owing to its high prevalence, morbidity, and death rates (Lv and Zhang, 2019). To manage CKD, it is crucial to promptly monitor kidney function and implement lifestyle changes and medications to prevent or delay disease progression (Johnson et al., 2013). The use of IoT-assisted technology and devices can significantly improve the management of CKD, given rapid advances in technology (Mamdiwar et al., 2021). Chronic kidney disease (CKD) is a significant public health concern, as it affects a substantial number of individuals worldwide, resulting in increased morbidity and mortality rates. IoT-supported technologies show promise in enhancing the treatment and management of CKD through increased patient involvement, enhanced communication between healthcare providers, and facilitation of remote monitoring (Albahri et al., 2021).

The Internet of Things (IoT) is an emerging, cutting-edge technology. The IoT revolution involves the integration of electronic engineering and computer science to create unique solutions. This technology is often used to create a network of physical objects that are equipped with sensors, software, hardware, and other technologies and are connected to the Internet for sharing or exchanging data with other connected objects or systems. In just a decade, IoT has had a significant impact on the healthcare industry. Healthcare is one of the many sectors to which the IoT offers its services. IoT plays a crucial role in healthcare settings to increase accuracy, productivity, and dependability. As the population grows, more people face health-related issues, and they need access to swift health services. IoT can be used to provide technological solutions for addressing this problem. This has led to the development of a multifaceted modern healthcare system, including its technological, social, and economic dimensions (Figure 4.1).

DOI: 10.1201/9781003469896-4

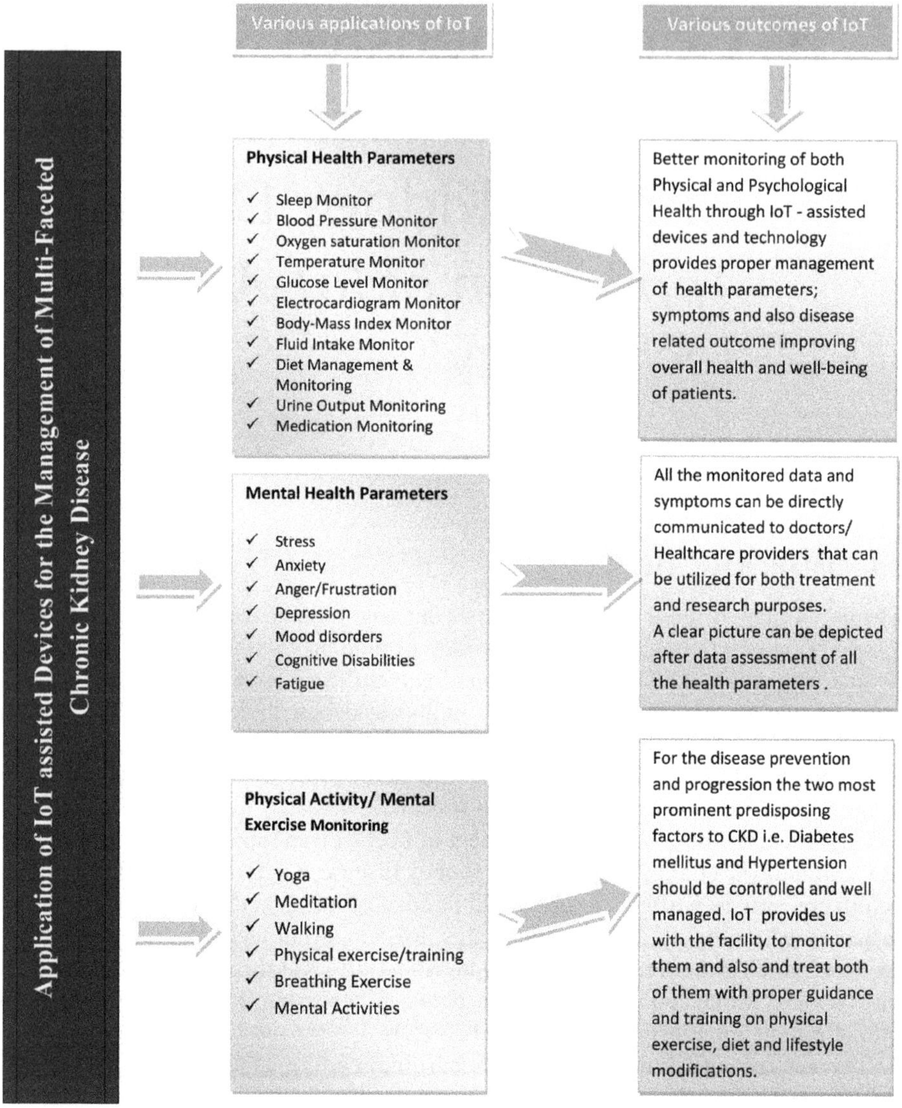

FIGURE 4.1 IoT-assisted devices and technology for monitoring and management of CKD.

This study sought to explore the role of IoT in healthcare and present advanced IoT services and applications. The paper's goal is to offer academics various paths for creating more effective and innovative IoT-based healthcare (Ravi et al., 2021). Devices aided by IoT for the management of CKD. IoT-based devices have the potential to transform the management of CKD by providing patients with timely data on their kidney function and general health status. Examples of such devices include the following: -

1. **Wearable devices:** Wearable technology, such as smartwatches, fitness trackers, and devices that rely on sensors, can monitor and track important health metrics such as heart rate, blood pressure, and blood sugar levels. In addition, these devices can identify the initial indicators of kidney damage and notify patients or their caregivers to take appropriate measures.
2. **Home monitoring devices:** Home monitoring devices, such as blood pressure monitors, scales, and glucometers, allow patients to monitor their health status in the comfort of their homes. Patients can transmit data from these devices to their healthcare providers, who can then adjust their treatment plans as necessary.
3. **Implantable devices:** Implantable devices such as kidney sensors can provide continuous monitoring of kidney function, allowing for early detection and intervention of complications.

Application of IoT-assisted technology in the management of CKD: IoT-assisted technology can be applied in the management of CKD in various ways, including:

1. **Telemedicine:** Home monitoring devices, including blood pressure monitors, scales, and glucometers, enable patients to monitor their health status in the comfort of their own homes by transmitting data to their healthcare providers, who can then adjust their treatment plans as needed.
2. **Personalized medicine:** IoT-assisted devices can collect real-time data on a patient's kidney function, allowing for the development of personalized treatment plans.
3. **Early detection of complications:** IoT-assisted devices can detect the early signs of kidney damage and other complications, allowing for early intervention and treatment.
4. **Self-management:** IoT-assisted devices can empower patients with CKD to take control of their health by providing real-time data on their health status and allowing them to monitor their progress.

4.2 LIMITATIONS

The reach of technology is expanding from developed to developing countries. In the Indian context, it is still in its infancy and requires more nurturing in order to be made available to the majority of the population suffering from not only CKD but also other chronic illnesses. While emerging countries see technological improvements, they also experience negative effects on immunity and health. Many people still cannot use technology because it is not cost-effective. There is still a lack of research in this area to fully understand the long-term impacts of adopting IoT-assisted technology, particularly when it comes to managing the healthcare of many people diagnosed with chronic diseases. Because CKD is an illness that renders patients very weak and vulnerable, utilizing IoT-assisted technology requires appropriate education, counseling, and training, none of which comes easily. Further investigation is required in this field of inquiry to improve knowledge and comprehension of all facets of chronic kidney disease, including complications and outcomes.

4.3 CONCLUSION

After evaluating the research related to the use of IoT-assisted tools and techniques for the management and treatment of chronic kidney disease (CKD), which is characterized by a loss of kidney function leading to the buildup of waste products in the body. Almost 10% of the global population is suffering from CKD. It is a fatal condition with high morbidity and mortality rates. As soon as possible after CKD is identified, renal function must be monitored, lifestyle changes should be done, and medication should be started in order to stop or delay the disease progression. As technology continues to advance rapidly and the Internet of Things (IoT) becomes more prevalent, there is great potential for IoT-assisted technologies and devices to detect diseases at an early stage. This can not only improve the chances of recovery but also slow down further loss or deterioration of kidney function. IoT can improve the treatment of CKD by better management of this multifaceted disease as it affects almost every part of a patient's life, including physiological, psychological, socio-emotional, and also financial domains of life. By giving patients access to real-time information about their kidney function and general health, IoT-assisted technology and devices have the potential to significantly enhance their disease outcomes. IoT-assisted devices can be used to support telemedicine, personalize treatment, identify issues at an early stage, and equip patients with the necessary tools to manage their own conditions. Examples of these devices include wearable home-monitoring systems and implantable sensors. The potential advantages of incorporating IoT technology in the management of CKD are substantial; however, additional research is necessary to gauge its effectiveness and impact. By promoting increased patient participation, enhancing patient-provider communication, and enabling remote monitoring, IoT-assisted technology has the potential to improve CKD management and treatment. However, to address the technical and usability challenges associated with implementing these technologies and to evaluate their long-term benefits and drawbacks, further research is required.

REFERENCES

Albahri, A. S., Alwan, J. K., Taha, Z. K., Ismail, S. F., Hamid, R. A., Zaidan, A. A., Albahri, O. S., Zaidan, B. B., Alamoodi, A. H., & Alsalem, M. A. (2021). IoT-based telemedicine for disease prevention and health promotion: State-of-the-art. *Journal of Network and Computer Applications*, 173, 102873.

Johnson, D. W., Atai, E., Chan, M., Phoon, R. K., Scott, C., Toussaint, N. D., Turner, G. L., Usherwood, T., & Wiggins, K. J. (2013). KHA-CARI guideline: Early chronic kidney disease: Detection, prevention and management. *Nephrology*, 18(5), 340–350.

Lv, J. C., & Zhang, L. X. (2019). Prevalence and disease burden of chronic kidney disease. In Bi-Cheng Liu, Hui-Yao Lan, Lin-Li Lv (eds). *Renal Fibrosis: Mechanisms and Therapies*, pp. 3–15.

Mamdiwar, S. D., Shakruwala, Z., Chadha, U., Srinivasan, K., & Chang, C. Y. (2021). Recent advances on IoT-assisted wearable sensor systems for healthcare monitoring. *Biosensors*, 11(10), 372.

Ravi, M. A., Shukla, R., & Mishra, R. (2021) Applications and services of Internet of Things (IoT) in healthcare: A comprehensive review.

Romagnani, P., Remuzzi, G., Glassock, R., Levin, A., Jager, K. J., Tonelli, M., Massy, Z., Wanner, C., & Anders, H. J. (2017). Chronic kidney disease. *Nature Reviews Disease Primers*, 3(1), 1–24.

5 Privacy and Security Aspects of AI Related to IoT in Healthcare Industry

Methods, Tools, Applications, and Open Challenges

Santhiya S., Jayadharshini P., Sharmila C., Abinaya N., Dinesh Kumar B., and Srinithi, A.

5.1 ASPECTS OF SECURITY AND PRIVACY IN IoT

The "Global network architecture" known as the "Internet of Things" connects real-world and digital things by utilizing data collection and communication tools. Today's Internet of Things (IoT) connects a variety of IP-based communication-capable devices, including sensors, to the Internet. IoT in the healthcare sector offers alternatives for distant surveillance, early detection, and medical treatment for institutionalized handicapped individuals. Persons or things can have sensors, actuators, RFID tags, and other IoT components attached to them. Caregiver access is made easier by such tools and tags. For example, IoT applications can read, recognize, locate, and control RFID tags on patients' or patients' personal equipment (Along with medical equipment). The potential exists for the healthcare sector to reconsider current practices done thanks to IoT, but doing so will be extremely tough. Connecting it will be difficult to manage all the different systems in the healthcare setting [1–5]. There will also constantly be inquiries concerning how these gadgets are secured in terms of security.

5.1.1 IoT Architecture

A number of layers make up the IoT architecture, starting with the edge technology layer at starting at the application layer at the bottom and finishing there. Two lower tiers help with data collection; however, the two higher there are layers in charge of using the app's' data.

DOI: 10.1201/9781003469896-5

5.1.2 Layers

The IoT architecture consists of four layers are depicted below in Figure 5.1 and Table 5.1. The following are the layers' roles, starting at the bottom.

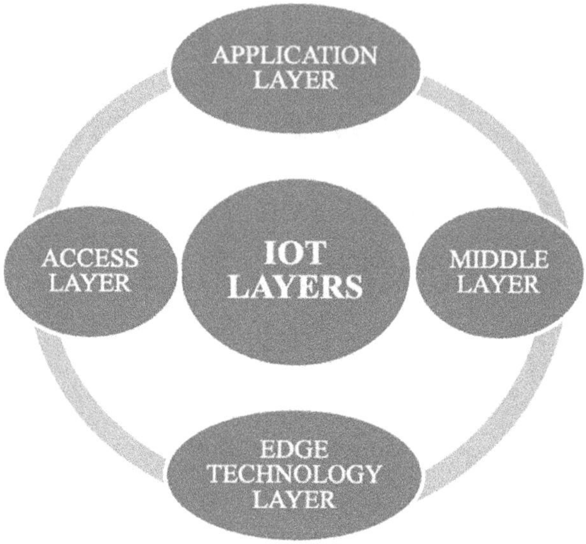

FIGURE 5.1 Layered architecture of IoT.

TABLE 5.1
Layers of IoT

Layers of IoT	Components of IoT	Tasks	Utilized Technology
Application layer	Application	Allow the disabled to see their health records and give them with care and support	Fog computing, cloud computing, home automation
Middleware layer	Eliminate discovery, access management, management of data	Enabling interaction between devices and applications	Lightweight, REST, OMA, EPC
Access gateway layer	Technology for communication	Wireless WAN: send data from devices or gateways.	Advance long-term evaluation, 4G, satellite system
Edge Technology layer	Physical things	Gather information about the environments of disabled users and keep track of them	
Identify them	Sensors, actuators, RFID		

5.1.2.1 Edge Technology Layer

Edge technology is sometimes called the perceiving layer. This is the lowest layer of the conventional architecture of IoT. Examples of the hardware that makes up this layer include cameras, RFID technology, wireless sensor networks (WSNs), intelligent terminals, and global positioning systems (GPS). It locates other intelligent devices nearby or picks up certain physical elements. These device elements provide communication, control, and actuation, such as with robots, as well as identification and information storage, such as with RFID tags, sensor networks, and embedded edge processors.

5.1.2.2 Gateway Layer for Access

The access gateway layer is sometimes referred to as the transport cover or network cover.

In this layer, in charge of processing data, which includes message publishing and subscribing message routing, and data transport. Using wireless and wired networks, Ethernet, GSM, WSN, and Wi-Max, it transfers information received between the middleware layer and the edge layer [6].

5.1.2.3 Intermediate Layer

It is a software platform that gives applications object abstraction. This layer is an essential component of the supporting architecture because it allows connections between sophisticated applications that were not originally intended to be coupled. Additionally, it provides a variety of services, such as Information discovery, data filtering, data aggregation, semantic data analysis, and access control (EPC or ONS) [7].

5.1.2.4 Layer of Applications

This is the upper layer in IoT Architecture. It is responsible for providing numerous applications to different IoT users. It has two below layers:

Data management sub-layer: It offers machine-to-machine (M2M) services, directory services, Data processing, cloud computing, quality of service (QoS), etc.

Application service sub-layer: This layer sits the layer above IoT apps and is incharge of interacting with end users and enterprise applications.

5.1.2.5 IoT's Place Medical Care

The deed of performing preventative or crucial procedures to improve a person's well-being is referred to in health care. You can achieve this through surgery, the use of medication, or other changes in lifestyle. Typically, a healthcare system composed of hospitals and doctors provides these services. IoT empowers healthcare workers to be more vigilant and actively engaged with their patients. So, with the help of IoT, physicians can be able to determine the patients' best course of treatment and achieve the desired results. IoT is crucial to the healthcare industry in a number of ways.

Mobile medical programs or wearables that enable patients to record their health data are another application of IoT in healthcare. Patients will be able to manage their own health more actively as a result. One of the industries that has embraced the "Internet of Things" the fastest is healthcare.

For individuals with chronic diseases, the elderly, and those who need ongoing care, utilizing IoT capabilities in medical apparatus increases the effectiveness and quality of the services provided.

5.1.2.6 IoT Security and Privacy Issues

Every day, more things are added to the "Internet of Things". Around 64 billion IoT devices could be in use worldwide by 2025. There has been a significant change in how daily tasks are carried out as a result of the increase in IoT devices. For instance, smart lighting may be able to lower your energy usage and electric bill. Additionally, the advantages of linked healthcare equipment have contributed to people's improvement in perceptions of their health. However, as the number of devices increases, the advantages come with noticeable concerns. The IoT ecosystem's expanding number of connected devices could provide security challenges because it will provide additional opportunities for hackers and cybercriminals to gain access. Every IoT application and system that supports the disabled is vulnerable to various security and privacy vulnerabilities.

5.1.2.7 Privacy of Patients Issues

An individual's personal electronic health record that complies with nationally accepted interoperability standards is known as a personal health record. PHR can be controlled, shared, and managed by the person and can be obtained from a variety of sources. The biggest security and privacy concern is maintaining PHRs of the patient's confidentiality because the PHRs immediately notified the health center.

5.1.2.8 Cyber-Attacks Threats on Privacy

Cyberattacks have the potential to introduce erroneous data into a system, seriously harming applications for IoT. It is essential to provide the appropriate degree of cyberattack protection for the disabled in smart home applications.

However, many of the IoT devices used in a smart home environment are resource-constrained, making it impossible to install typical security solutions.

5.1.3 Data Privacy and Data Eavesdropping

Patients' health information, particularly that of the disabled, is often held under legal responsibilities of secrecy and is only accessible to the designated carers. Data theft from storage and listening in on them as they travel via wireless networks must be avoided. For instance, a well-known Internet of Things insulin delivery and insulin level monitoring system uses consisting of wireless communication lines, which are routinely utilized to conduct privacy assaults. By violating their privacy, data eavesdropping could harm the disabled. Utilizing public key encryption will increase data secrecy (PKI). Data encryption is made more efficient by PKI since it may establish a high level of confidence while transmitting information in a risky setting.

5.1.4 Security Issues for Applications

The Internet of Things (IoT) with machine-to-machine communication capabilities has developed from the Internet for PCs. Making IoT affordable and expanding the range of supported devices is crucial if it is to become widely used. Before realizing the goal of greater IoT adoption, there are significant technical and security challenges that must be resolved. Energy, wireless communication, scalability, security, and other technical difficulties with IoT exist.

5.1.5 Methods to Overcome Privacy and Security Issues

Security breaches may occur as a result of carelessness or ignorance. Your personnel, Patients, regulatory authorities, or cloud service providers neglecting to concentrate more on a potential issue could all be held responsible if your organization is the target of the hacker assault through an issue with a linked device. On an organizational level, however, a preventive strategy is most effective. Communities in healthcare have come to terms with the notion it will be IoT play a role in their upcoming. They are aware that digitizing and simplifying the exchange of health information will increase their efficiency and save them a lot of money. Manufacturers and suppliers of IoT devices can adopt a number of fundamental security measures, such as encryption and secure booting.

Make sure that using a device is restricted; the software is provided to the apparatus only after verification, in addition to device-to-device connectivity is kept under observation. Make sure that there is sufficient access controls in position that restrict unapproved access to IoT devices, networks, and data. Before going into production, the IoT device's security should be tested, and security should be tracked all the way through the device's life. Create an environment of security where staff are educated to spot weaknesses.

5.1.5.1 Ensure System Protection

By offering network segmentation and securing each subnet on its level, healthcare organizations minimize potential network security breaches.

Even if data is intercepted by hackers, network administrators can manage the stream of information Use encryption methods between each network segment to prevent evidence from being deciphered.

5.1.5.2 Data Encryption

Data encryption is included in the IoT for healthcare, as well as methods to overcome privacy and security issues. Connected devices typically employ both symmetric and asymmetric lightweight cryptography methods, and parties typically exchange encryption keys before data flow. IoT sensors today typically include encryption keys for creating a secure HTTP channel between devices and consumers.

5.1.5.3 Tools

The various tools used in Healthcare IoT's are,

- Online patient observation,
- Controlling blood sugar,
- Hand hygiene observation,
- Consumable sensors,
- Automated surgery.

5.1.5.4 Online Patient Observation

The most prevalent use of IoT gadgets in healthcare is online patient observation. IoT gadgets can automatically assemble health data obtained from patients who are not physically present at a hospital, including temperature, blood pressure, heart rate, and more, removing the requirement that patients travel to the doctors or pick it up themselves. Any time an IoT device gathers patient information, it sends the information using software programmed, so that patients and/or healthcare providers can examine it. In order to make treatment recommendations or produce alerts, algorithms may be employed to analyze the data. IoT sensor that notices a sufferer's exceptionally minimal heartbeat, for instance, may sound a warning so that medical personnel can take action.

Making sure these IoT devices collect personal information is private and safe is a significant barrier for remote patient monitoring equipment.

5.1.5.5 Controlling Blood Sugar

Controlling blood sugar devices minimizes the necessity of maintaining manual records and can warn when patients' blood sugar amounts are troublesome.

Designing an Internet of Things glucose monitoring gadget that:

a. It's compact and adequate to allow continuous monitoring with no disruption for the patients
b. It does not require regular recharging due to its low electricity consumption.

5.1.5.6 Hand Hygiene Observation

In order to reduce the risk of spreading illness, there hasn't always been an effective way to make sure that staff members and patients in a medical facility properly clean their hands. IoT devices are now widely used by hospitals and other healthcare facilities to recall people before hand washing entering patient spaces. Even suggestions on the best ways to sterilize to lessen a specific threat to certain suffers might be provided by the devices. The fact that these tools can simply serve as a reminder for people to wash their hands—rather than really doing the action—is a serious drawback. However, evidence indicates that these gadgets can lower hospital infection rates by more than 60%.

5.1.5.7 Consumable Sensors

The process of gathering information internal to the human body is often untidy and also quite eruptive. It is substantially less invasive to gather data on the digestive system and other systems when using consumable sensors. For example, they reveal information about stomach PH levels or assist in determining the cause of gastrointestinal bleeding. These gadgets need to be tiny enough to be swallowed with ease. Additionally, they must have a means of annihilation or neatly exit the body on their own. Many companies are operating diligently on absorbable sensors that meet these specifications.

5.1.5.8 Automated Surgery

Through the placement of tiny Internet-connected robots inside human anatomy, surgeons may perform difficult surgeries in the case difficult to do use human hands. Furthermore, minimally invasive automated surgery carried out by tiny IoT gadgets can reduce the necessary incision size prior to surgery, making the procedure less invasive and hastening patient recovery. These tools need to be diminutive, dependable, and sufficient to perform surgery with minimal interruption. Additionally, they must be able to understand intricate situations occurring interior of bodies to enable decision-making regarding what to do next throughout a procedure. However, the application of Smart robots in surgery shows that these challenges can be surmounted.

5.2 WHAT EFFECTS WILL IoT HAVE ON THE HEALTHCARE INDUSTRY?

Numerous IoT applications, including telemedicine and telehealth, are used in the healthcare industry for both health monitoring and treatment. Applications could include long-distance health care and education delivery using medical technology and the Internet. Medical devices, which can be implanted, injectable, or ingestible, as well as wearable or non-wearable, can enable remote monitoring of a patient's vital signs, chronic conditions, or other health and wellness indicators. Thirty-six wireless medical devices can be utilized for remote monitoring and care ,as well as in hospital settings, saving patients from frequent or prolonged hospital stays. According to several analysts, improvements in IoT applications for the healthcare sector will be crucial for offering the aging U.S. population accessible, high-quality treatment.

5.3 WHAT ARE THE BIGGEST PRIVACY AND SECURITY CONCERNS WITH A "THINGSINTERNET"

Cyberattacks may also threaten privacy, allowing access to and exfiltration of a person's identifying information or other sensitive information. For instance, access to a wearable gadget could allow the exfiltration of information on the wearer's whereabouts, activities, or even health. Questions about ownership, processing, and use of such data are included in privacy issues, in addition to the issue of whether security precautions are sufficient to thwart such invasions.

Large volumes of data about people and organizations may be generated and retained by both commercial companies and governments as the deployment of IoT objects increases.

5.4 CHALLENGES

The challenges faced in IoT's are:

5.4.1 Scalability

Scalability is an important factor in the medical industry. To put it another way, it is a system's capacity to adapt to evolving needs and adjust to developments that will be more significant in the future. However, it appears to be a challenging because the offered ways were generally applied in confined contexts.

5.4.2 Standardization and Compatibility

The capacity of patients and smart objects to exchange information and resources depends in large part on the interoperability of IoT. The main obstacle to interoperability is creating stable open-source frameworks. To build horizontal platforms with operability, programmability, and communication between hardware, operating systems, and software, a set of standards must be developed. without being worried about the model or the product's maker or model.

5.4.3 Mobility

One of the biggest difficulties in IoT. In IoT healthcare systems, mobility speaks of the capacity to make use of network assistance so that patients can connect to the gateway whenever and wherever they choose Additionally, mobility is required to improve service quality, make information accessible to all regardless of users' locations, and make the network fault-tolerant. A mobility protocol is necessary and dependable to reduce end-to-end delays, packet losses, and network failures under any circumstances because provisioning is crucial in the healthcare industry. Therefore, mobility presents an intriguing research problem.

5.4.4 Actual Testbed Setting

Only 24% of the examined research used real testbeds, while the remainder used simulation tools to test the IoT concepts that were recommended; this needs to be applied in real contexts. Real testbed implementation is difficult as a result. Some of the common challenges faced in IoT are depicted in Figure 5.2.

5.5 SUMMARY

IoT, or the Internet of Things, significant strides recently, and these innovations hold enormous promise for healthcare solutions. However, IoT healthcare applications face numerous security and privacy concerns. This Paper discusses "Internet of Things", its layered architecture, and the healthcare sector. It offers the idea of focusing on privacy as the key where security and privacy meet. It also explains security and privacy services.

IoT will become the core component of the Future Internet. It serves as a link between the physical and digital worlds. Before using IoT, there are numerous privacy and information security issues that need to be taken into account. To make sure the items can coexist in a smooth and nonaggressive contexts equally effectively, the pace of development must increase as objects get smarter. Although many other IoT-related topics, including applications, architecture, and many others, were explored in this article, the security and privacy concerns were given the most attention.

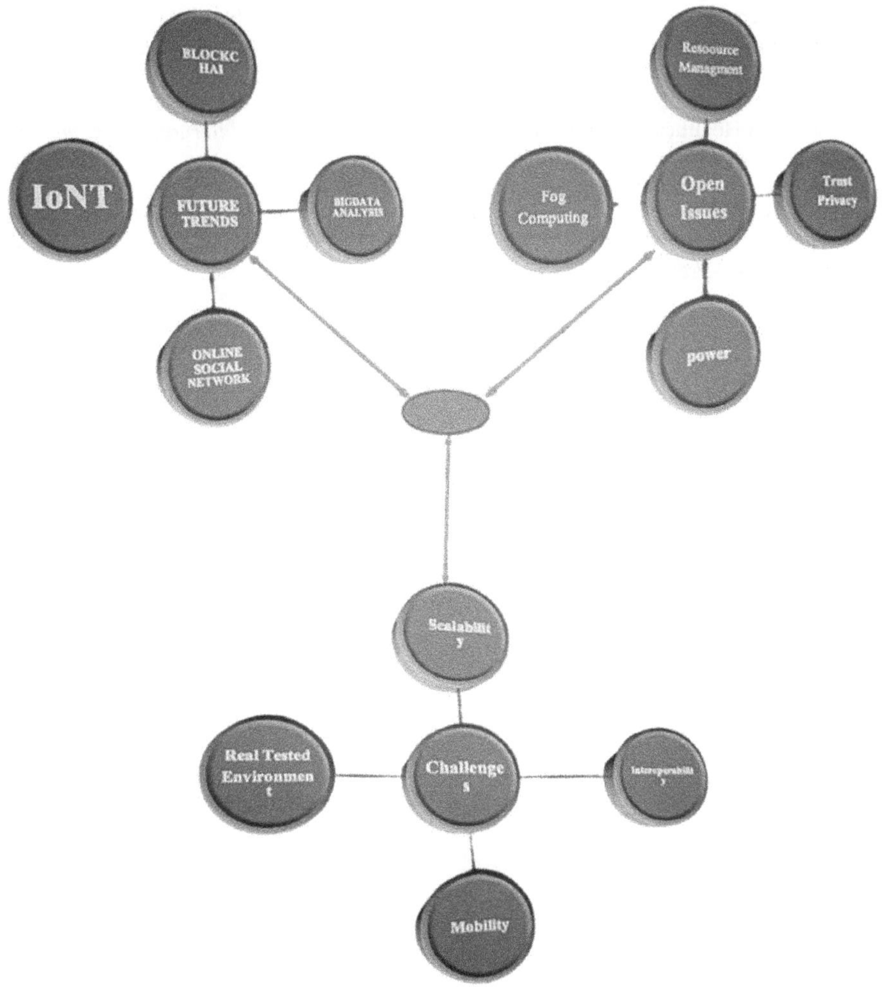

FIGURE 5.2 Challenges faced in IoT.

REFERENCES

1. D. Giusto, A. Iera, G. Morabito, and L. Atzori, "An Overview of Privacy and Security Issues inthe Internet of Things," In Daniel Giusto, Antonio Iera, Giacomo Morabito, Luigi Atzori (eds). *The Internet of Things*, 1st Ed., Springer, New York, 2010, pp. 389–395.
2. C. M. Medaglia and A. Serbanati, "An Overview of Privacy and Security Issues in the Internet of Things," In *Proceedings of 20th Tyrrhenian Workshop on Digital Communications*, Italy, 2010, pp. 389–395.
3. Z. Qian, Y. Wang, X. Wang, and S. Zhu, "M/I Adaptation Layer Network Protocol for IoT Basedon 6LoWPAN," In Yongheng Wang, Xiaoming Zhang (eds). *The Internet of Things*, Springer, Changsha, Aug. 19, 2012, pp. 208–215.

4. K. Finkenzeller, "Known Attacks on RFID Systems, Possible Countermeasures and Upcoming Standardisation Activities," In *5th European Workshop on RFID Systems and Technologies*, Nov. 2009, pp. 1–31.
5. V. M. Rohokale, N. R. Prasad, and R. Prasad, "A Cooperative Internet of Things (IoT) for Rural Healthcare Monitoring and Control," In *IEEE 2nd International Conference on Wireless Communication*, Chennai, Feb. 2011, pp. 1–6.
6. Wireless Communication for IoT. Last access June 16, 2015.
7. T. Harriet, "How the 'Internet of Things' Could Be Fatal," Mar. 4, 2016; L. Ayala, "Cybersecurity for Hospitals and Healthcare Facilities - A Guide to Detection and Prevention," Fredericksburg, VA.

6 Ontology-Based Expert System for Lung Cancer Disease Diagnosis

Nadiminti Venkata Ramana Murty

6.1 INTRODUCTION OF SEMANTIC WEB MODELING FOR LUNG CANCER PREDICTIVE SYSTEM

Artificial Intelligence-based expert system design is very useful. A computer system that can behave like a human expert and solve problems in a particular domain is termed an Expert System [1]. The main units of an Expert system are GUI, Inference Engine, Working Memory, and Knowledge Base. The general architecture of an Expert system is shown in Figure 6.1.

Figure 6.1 depicts the interaction mechanism of the user with the system through the GUI. Knowledge Base is developed as a set of rules and facts. Inference Engine helps to derive new knowledge from experience [2]. It will be supported by an expert interface to update the as when new knowledge comes into existence on the subject.

6.2 SEMANTIC WEB

Semantic Web is an extension topic to the World Wide Web (www), which delivers a simple and easier way to find, share, reuse, and combine information. It uses XML (eXtensible Markup Language) and RDF (Resource Description Framework) to represent information. This section comprises of design and development of a Semantic Web-based predictive system based on ontology [3]. The general architecture of the Semantic Web is shown in Figure 6.2 [4,5].

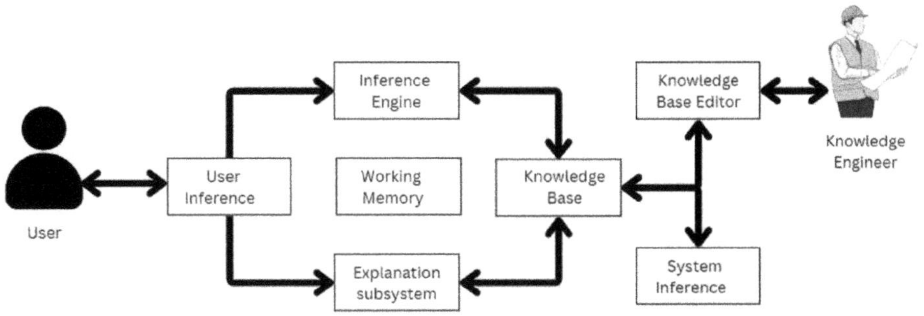

FIGURE 6.1 The architecture of an expert system.

DOI: 10.1201/9781003469896-6

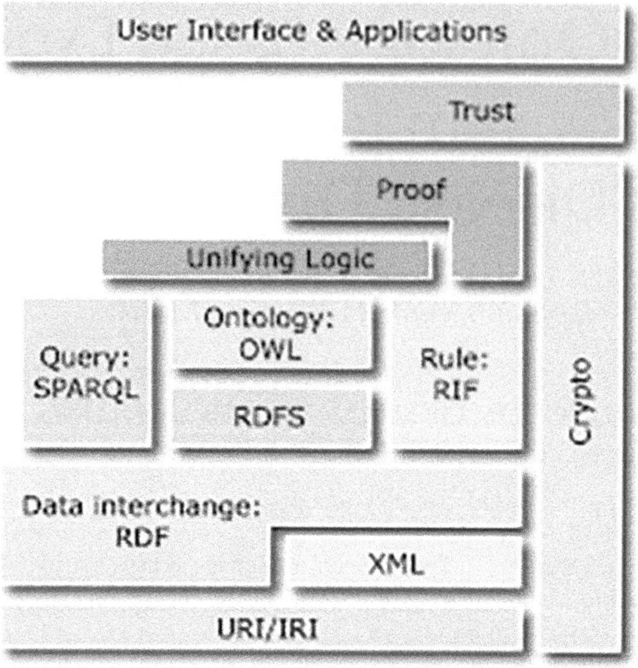

FIGURE 6.2 The architecture of semantic web.

6.3 ONTOLOGIES IN PREDICTIVE SYSTEMS

Ontology is a set of concepts and categories used for knowledge encoding in the form of common vocabularies and which can be made useful to show their properties and the associations between them.

Diagnosing lung cancer diseases in their early stages is always helpful and determines the best treatment. Building an ontology-based predictive system is used to identify the status of the disease and, thereby, the treatment of the patient [1]. The general view of a Predictive system based on Ontology is shown in Figure 6.3. A Predictive system model presented in Figure 6.3 contains four major block components [6,7]:

1. **Ontology questions**
2. **SWRL Rules**
3. **System Components &**
4. **Disease Level Treatment Procedures**

6.3.1 Ontologies Development

Figure 6.4 shows the general procedure to develop an Ontology. The Ontological Modeling system will govern the concepts and terminology of a given problem and then distinguish the problem field. The working procedure of Ontological modeling is explained in the subsequent section [8–11].

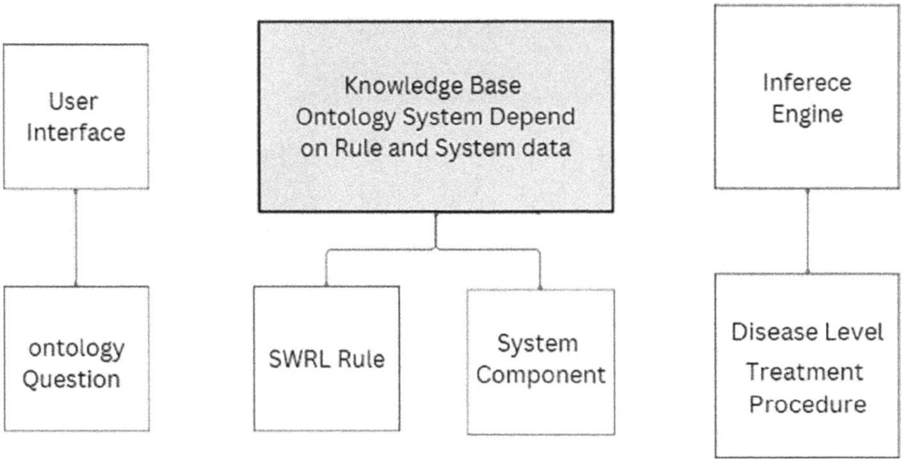

FIGURE 6.3 Predictive system model based on ontology.

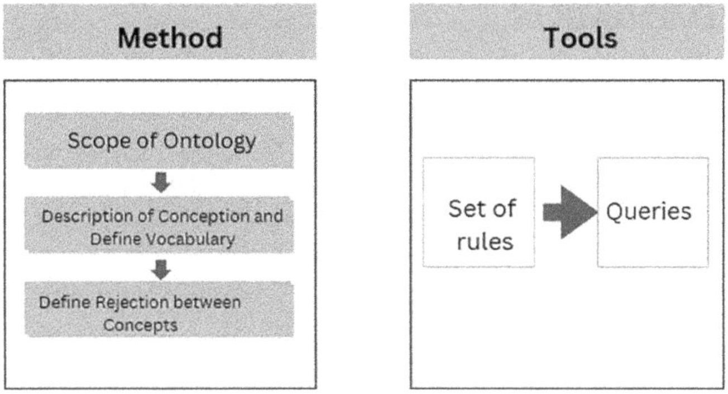

FIGURE 6.4 Ontology development procedure.

6.3.2 Ontology Development for Lung Cancer Predictive System

Lung cancer is most commonly attacked a disease that causes death worldwide. Besides, all researchers agree that improving the life-expectancy depends on the initial level diagnosis of the illness. The proposed system will assist the expert in the early prediction and diagnosis of lung cancer and thereby improve the rate of survival of the patients.

The semantic web predictive system supports the user/patient to know his/her level of the disease and helps in suggesting the experts (Doctors) diagnose lung cancer correctly within the stipulated time. Here, Ontology-based knowledge system evaluates the patient situation based on SWRL rules developed based on some questions and rules recommended by an oncology expert [12]. The architecture of the Semantic Web-based Lung Cancer Predictive System is given in Figure 6.5. The implementation details of the components are presented in Section 6.4 [10,11,13].

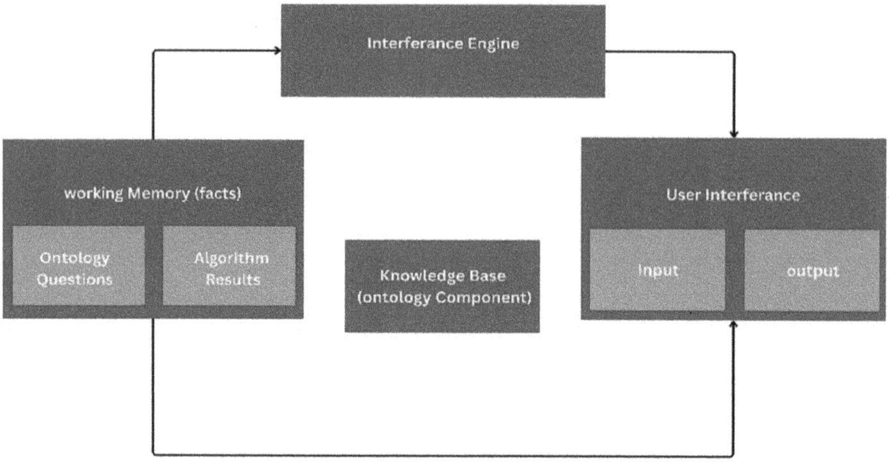

FIGURE 6.5 Implementation of Lung Cancer Predictive System.

6.4 IMPLEMENTATION

Implementation of the proposed Semantic Web-Based Predictive System for Lung Cancer Diagnosis is explained in the following subsections. All components of the proposed system are implemented using PROTEGE 4.0 Editor, which is the Application Programming Interface (API) of Java, to form the knowledge base with the use of a Plug-in type construction [12]. This program supports the depiction, imagining, and variations in the ontologies [10,11,14,15].

The major features of this tool are

a. User-friendly Interface
b. Several useful plug-ins
c. Enable the designer to edit the contents in the GUI itself without writing programming code.

6.4.1 User Interface Implementation

This component consists of a Graphics User Interface (GUI) that enables users to enter data. The same interface can also be used for knowledge acquisition from experts. A new patient object can also be added to this semantic system, as shown in Figure 6.6. Here Patient Name, Age, Gender, Smokes or not is provided [16,17].

6.4.2 Working Memory

The second module represents working memory, which contains two sub-modules. The first sub-module is ontology questions, which collect information such as name, age, and symptoms from the user interface. This will enable to the generation of ontology classes to develop "a patient object" [18]. The second part of the working

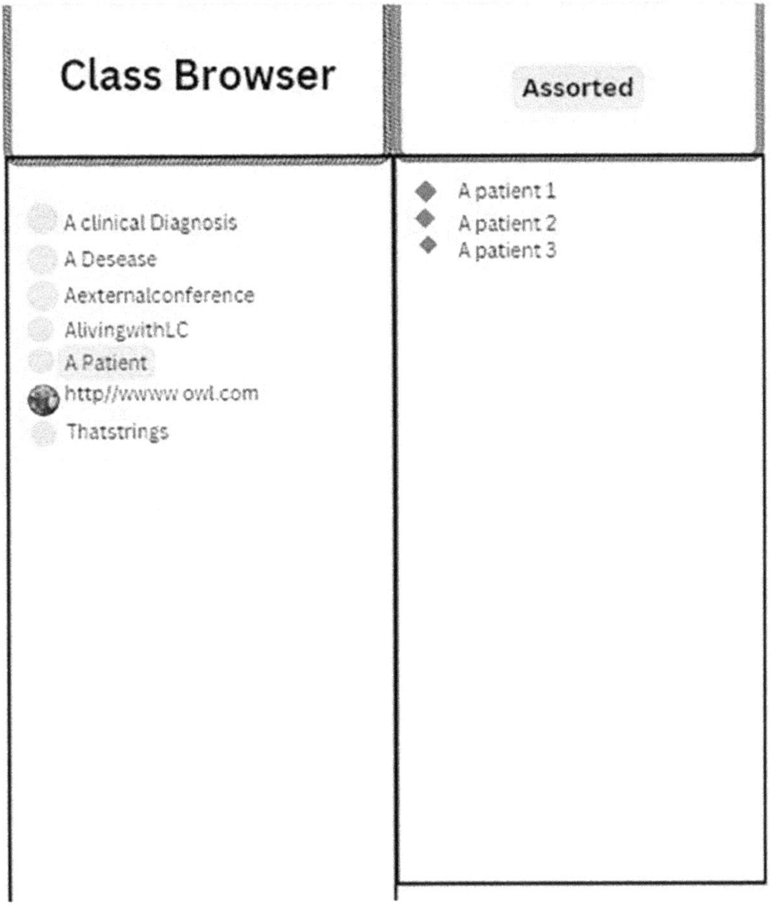

FIGURE 6.6 User interface.

memory consists of textual data, numeric data, and imprecise data components. The screenshots are shown in Figure 6.7. Illustrate the working memory components.

6.4.3 Knowledge Base

The third component of the proposed predictive system is the knowledge base, which stores classes, objects, and their corresponding relationships in the form of SWRL rules [19]. The web ontologies related to data property and object property are shown in the form of a screenshot represented in Figures 6.8 and 6.9.

6.4.4 Inference Engine

The fourth component is the Inference Engine (IE). The proposed system depends on the JESS engine to suggest the best treatment to the patient, as per the decision given

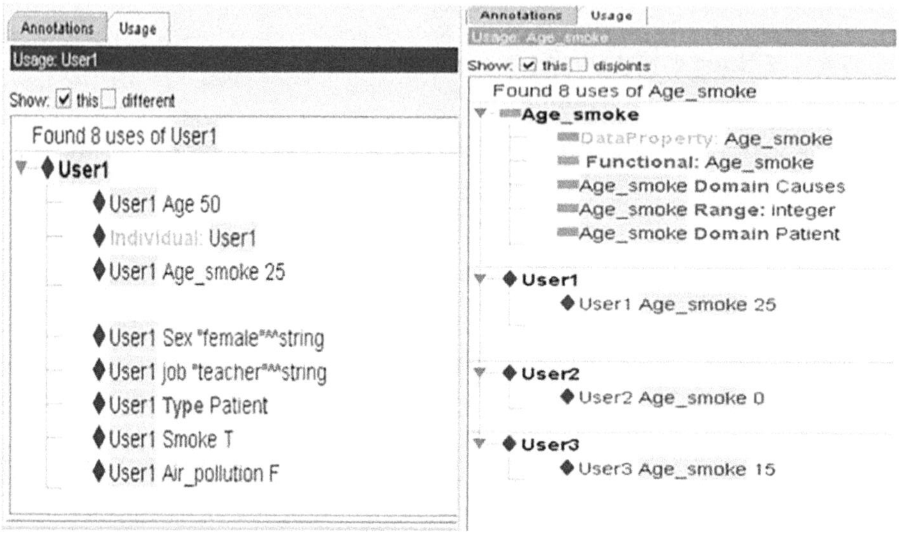

FIGURE 6.7 Working memory.

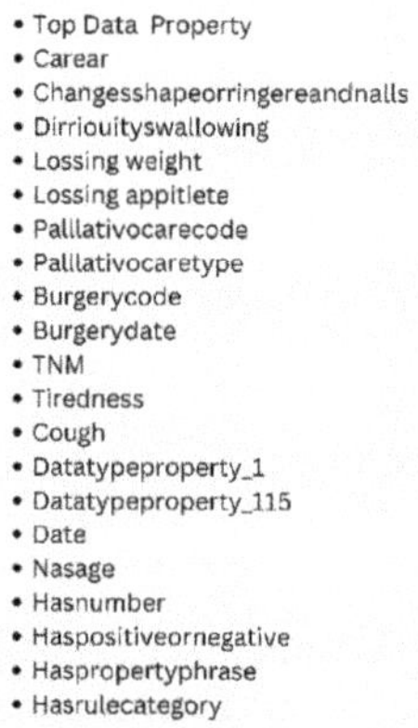

FIGURE 6.8 Data property.

by the rules. IE computes the patient status depending on the symptoms entered by the user by inferencing the SWRL rules stored in the knowledge base and generating its recommendations.

In the Ontology model, the data that is expressible can be collected from the relation, but there is a need to collect the data that is not expressible from the ontology language [20].

In case the existing SWRL rules are not sufficient to deduce conclusions, the IE may import additional information from OWL, operated by JESS (JAVA Expert System Shell) The procedure is described in Table 6.1.

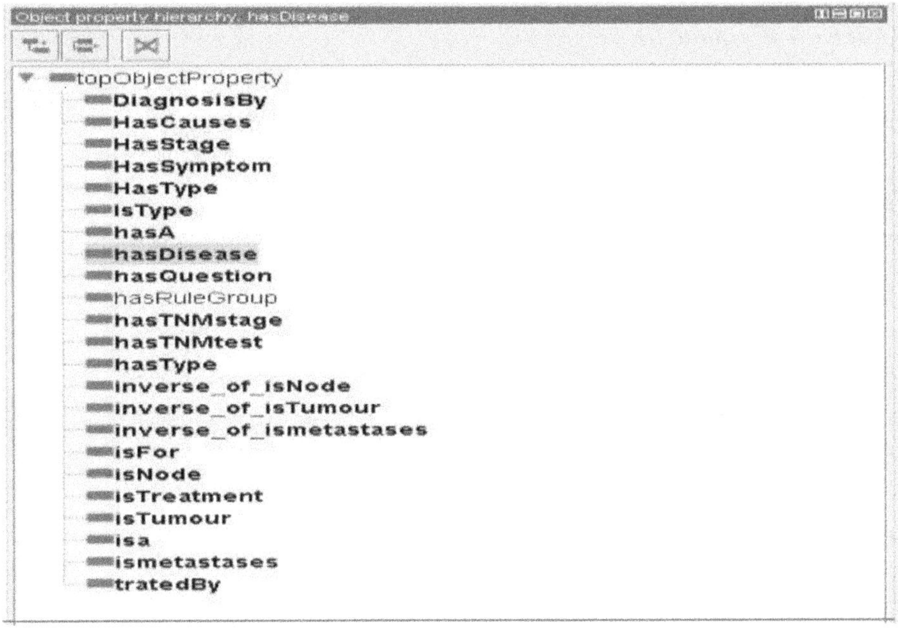

FIGURE 6.9 Object property.

TABLE 6.1
SWRL Rules

Rule Name	Expiration
http://www.owl-ontologies.com/Determine_NSCLC_type2	Patient(?p)^isNode(?p,?n) sqwrl:equal(?n,N2) ^isTumour(?p,?t)^sqwr:equal(?t,T3)^ismetastases(?p,?m) ^sqwr:equal(?m,M1a)→LargCellCaricnoma(?p)
http://www.owl-ontologies.com/Ontologylungcancer12.owl#IF_algorithm_Result_True	Patient(?p)^AlgorithmResult(?a)°sqwrl:equal (?a,AlgorithmResul2)→hasDisease(?a,Sclcl)
http://www.owl-ontologies.com/Ontologylungcancer12.owl#if_hasSymptom_and_algrithemResult(true)_treatmentWith_bronchoscopy	Patient(?p)^AlgorithmResult(?a)°sqwrl:equal(?a,true) ^HasSyptom(?p,?s)→Bonchoscopy(?p)
http://www.owl-ontologies.com/Ontologyluncancer12.owl#if_TNM(true)_an_diagnosisBy(surgicalBiopsy)_treatmentBy_chemotherpy	Patient(?p)^TNM(?p,?k)°sqwl:equal(?k,true)^SurgicalBiopsy(?o)→Chemotheraphy(?p)
http://www.owl-ontologies.com/Ontologylungcancer12.owl#determine_first_symptoms_if_Questienl_answer(true)_coughQ1	Qeustion(?q)^cough(?q,?y)°swrl:equal(?y,true)→Symptom(cough)

(Continued)

TABLE 6.1 (*Continued*)
SWRL Rules

Rule Name	Expiration
http://www.owl-ontologies.com/ Ontologylungcancer12. owl#Diagnosis_lungcancer_by_ctscan	Patient(?p)^CTScan(?c)^Symptom(?s)^HasSymptom (?p,?s)→DiagnoisBy(?p,?c)
http://www.owl-ontologies.com/ Ontologylungcancer12. owl#stage_lungcancer_dependeon_TNM	Patient(?e)^TNMStagingSystem(?w)^sqwrl:notEmpt y(?e,?w)→HasSage(?e,?w)
http://www.owl-ontologies.com/ Ontologylungcancer12. owl#symptom_and_stage_to_livingwithlc	ungcancer(?p)^Symptom(?s)^HasStage(?p,?t)°sqwrl: equal(?t,A1_6)→LivingWithLC(?p)
http://www.owl-ontologies.com/ Ontologylungcancer12. owl#diagnosis_diseasBY_and_hasSymptom_ determin_lungcancer	Patient(?p)^DiagnosisBy(?p,?d)°sqwrl:equal(?d,Dian oses_5)^HasSymptom(?p,?s)^sqwrl:equal(?s,Sympt om_8)→Lungcancer(?p)
http://www.owl-ontologies.com/ Ontologylungcancer12. owl#Determin_NSCLC_typel	Patient(?p)^isNode(?p,?n)°sqrl:equal(?n,N1)^isTumo ur(?p,?t)^sqwrl:equal(?t,T2)^ismetastases(?p,?m)^sq wr:equal(?m,M0)---adenocarcinoma(?p)
http://www.owl-ontologies.com/ Ontologylungcancer12. owl#Determine_NSCLC_type3	Patient(?p)^isNode(?p,?n)°sqwrlequal(?n,N3)^isTum our(?p,?t)^sqwrl:equal(?t,T4)^ismetastases(?p,?m)^s qwrl:equal(?m,M1b)→SquamousCellCaricnoma(?p)
http://www.owl-ontologies.com/ Ontologylungcancer12. owl#patient_has_NSCLC_and_hasage_need_ pallitativecare	Patient(?p)^NONSmallcellLC(?n)^has Age(?p,?age)° sqwrlgreatet(?age,50)→PalliativeCare(?p)
http://www.owl-ontologies.com/ Ontologylungcancer12. owl#work_in_some_place_to_have_ hungcancer_Rule-carear	Patient(?r)^cough(?r,?y)°sqwrl:equal(?y,true)→lungc ancer(?r)
http://www.owl-ontologies.com/ Ontologylungcancer12. owl#tretment_patient_by_Rule-surgry	Patient(?f)^isTumour(?f,?o)^ismeastases(?f,?u)^isNo e(?f,?e)°sqwrl:equal(?o,Tla)^sqwrl:equal(?u,N0)^ sqwrl:equal(?e,M0)→isTreatment(?f,Surgry)

6.4.5 SWRL Rules

Rules can be created in Ontology with the help of Semantic Web Rule Language (SWRL) based on the patient's medical information. The rules generated can be used to determine the relationships among individuals and classes. Like the rule of surgery depends on the following [21,22], A typical expert system rule and the corresponding SWRL rule are given below.

6.4.5.1 Expert System Rule

If Metastases are Zero (0), Node I is Zero (0,) and the Tumour is T1a, then the expert system decision is the disease may be small cell cancer, and the suggested diagnosis for the medical treatment is surgery.

6.4.5.2 SWRL Rule

If Metastases(?f,?u) A isTumour(?f,?o) A Patient(?f) A isNode(?f,?e) ° sqwrl:equal(?o, T1a) A sqwrl:equal(?u, N0) A sqwrl:equal(?e, M0) → isTreatment(?f, Surgery)

Similarly, the remaining SWRL rules are generated corresponding to expert system rules. In the next phase patient consolidated report is to be generated based on the inference mechanism outlined in Section 6.4.4. The results are presented in Figure 6.10.

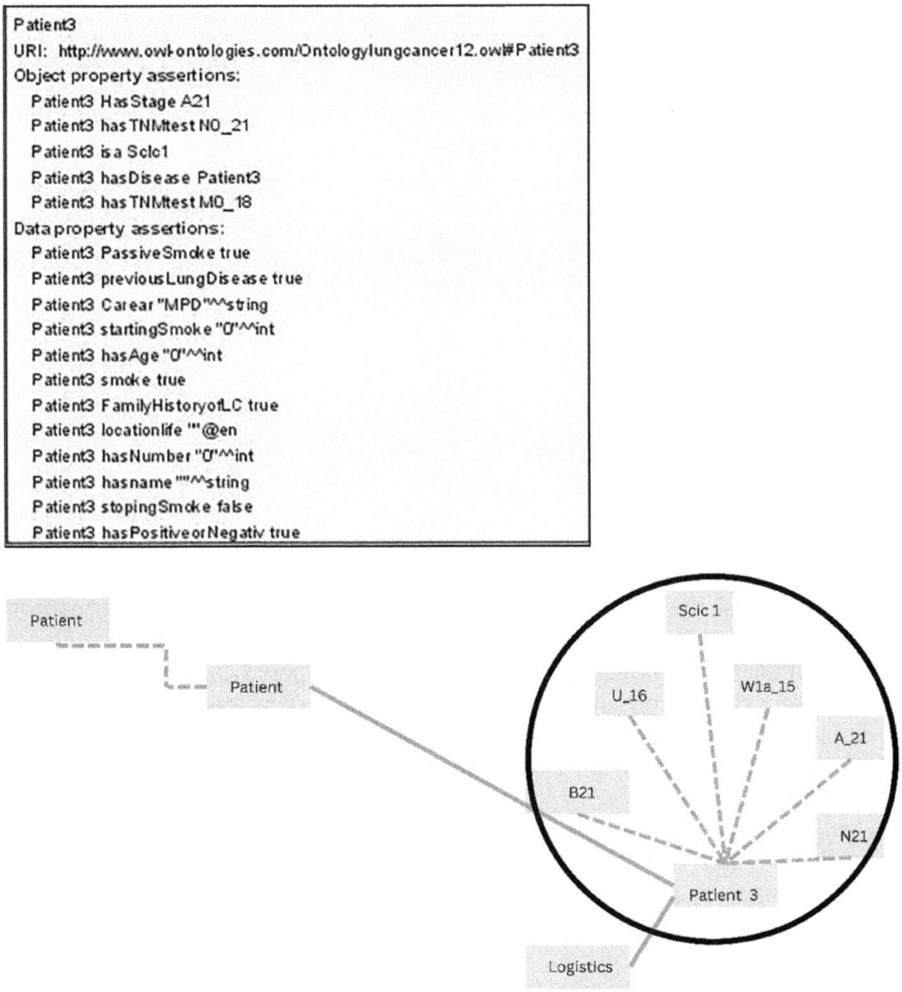
Patient3
URI: http://www.owl-ontologies.com/Ontologylungcancer12.owl#Patient3
Object property assertions:
Patient3 HasStage A21
Patient3 hasTNMtest N0_21
Patient3 is a Sclc1
Patient3 hasDisease Patient3
Patient3 hasTNMtest M0_18
Data property assertions:
Patient3 PassiveSmoke true
Patient3 previousLungDisease true
Patient3 Carear "MPD"^^string
Patient3 startingSmoke "0"^^int
Patient3 hasAge "0"^^int
Patient3 smoke true
Patient3 FamilyHistoryofLC true
Patient3 locationlife ""@en
Patient3 hasNumber "0"^^int
Patient3 hasname ""^^string
Patient3 stopingSmoke false
Patient3 hasPositiveorNegativ true

FIGURE 6.10 Patient instances.

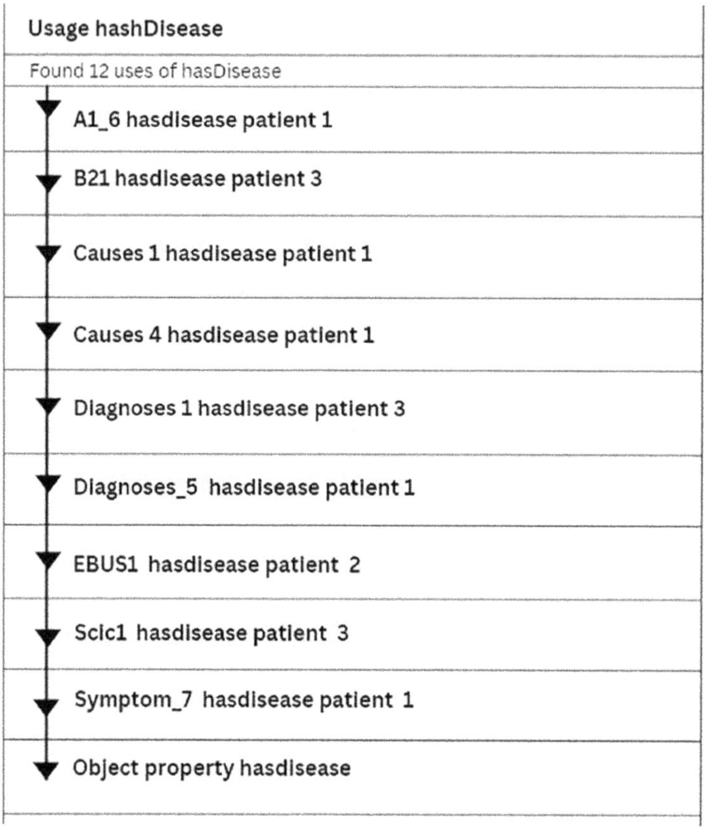

FIGURE 6.11 Has_disease property.

The object relations among various objects are presented in Figure 6.11. Here the object relationship among the object concerning **'has_disease'** is the illness property for the individual class of the patient [23]. This example of the defined property is used in this design.

A set of queries and rules are created to test the proposed Ontology. The results of the present system are validated by comparing the system-generated outputs with doctor annotations. Figure 6.12 'Query of Ontology System [24], retrieves the patient ID that has the result positive concerning the disease [10,11,25–26].

6.5 RESULTS AND DISCUSSIONS

In this section, lung cancer ontology and working procedure of the semantic web predictive system are described in terms of screenshots depicted in Figures 6.13–6.21. The Lung Cancer Predictive System [27] Ontology is derived by using Protege 4.0 Editor. The Screenshot generated is shown in Figure 6.13.

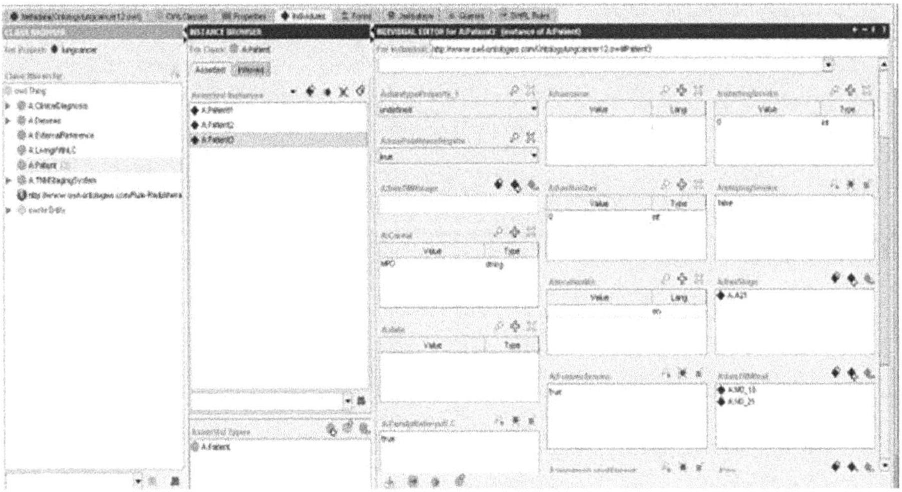

FIGURE 6.12 Query of Ontology System.

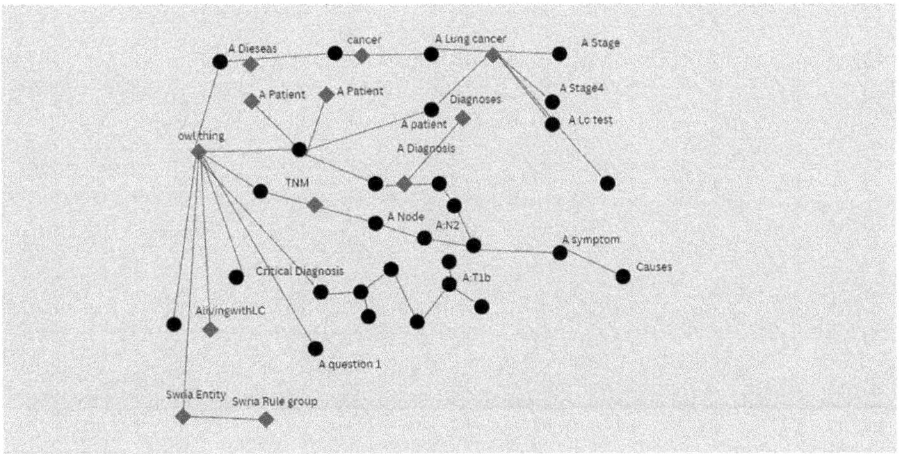

FIGURE 6.13 The Lung Cancer Predictive System Ontology.

6.5.1 Working Procedure of the Present System

The working procedure of the present system is described in the following steps.

Step 1: On the Homepage, click the "Enter Symptoms" button. Choose the Checkboxes of Symptoms list and click on the submit button.

Step 2: Select the Checkboxes which are appropriate to the symptoms

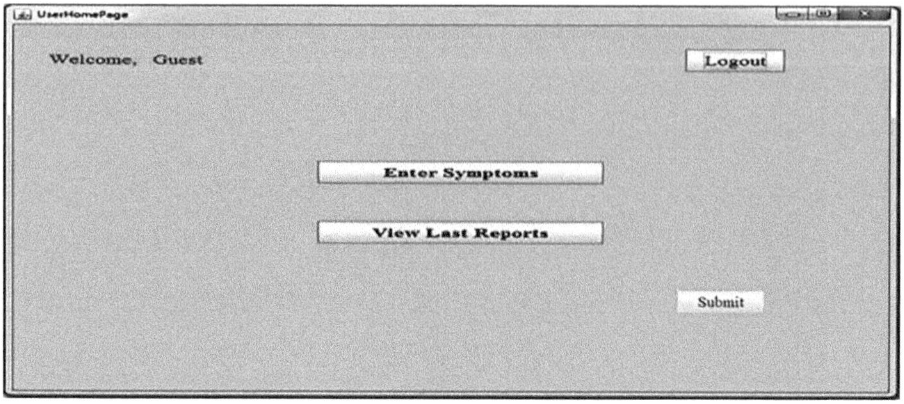

FIGURE 6.14 Homepage for entering symptoms.

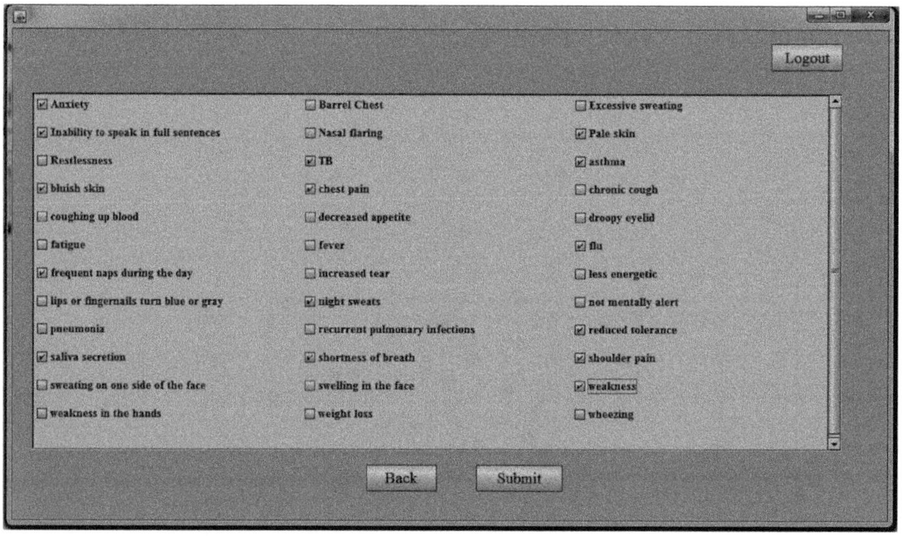

FIGURE 6.15 Selecting checkboxes for choosing symptoms.

Step 3: The Entered Symptoms represent the disease name screen
Step 4: Choosing the severity of the symptoms to increase the optimization of the results
Step 5: Displaying the Disease Name
Step 7: Showing the Last Reports

6.5.2 Working Procedure for Updating the Present System

When a user (Expert/admin) desires to update the knowledge base he has to open the following web page. It has the following links [28–30].

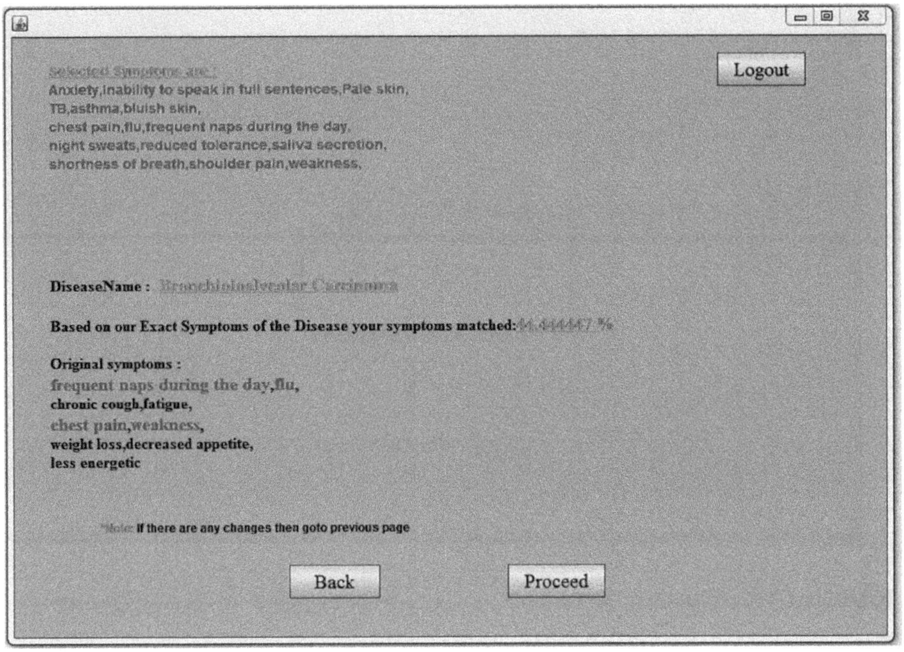

FIGURE 6.16 Displaying disease name.

(a)
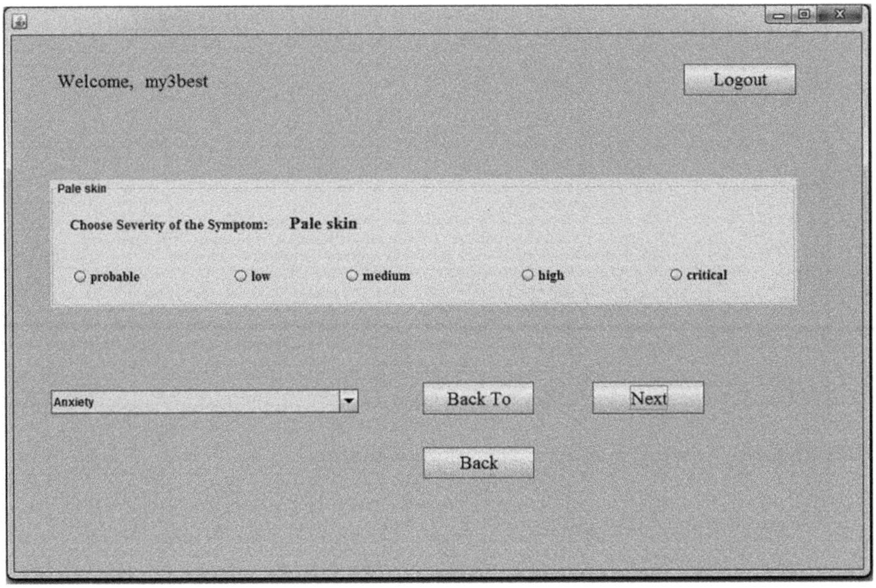

FIGURE 6.17 (a) Choosing severity of the symptom. (b) Choosing severity of the symptom.

(Continued)

(b)

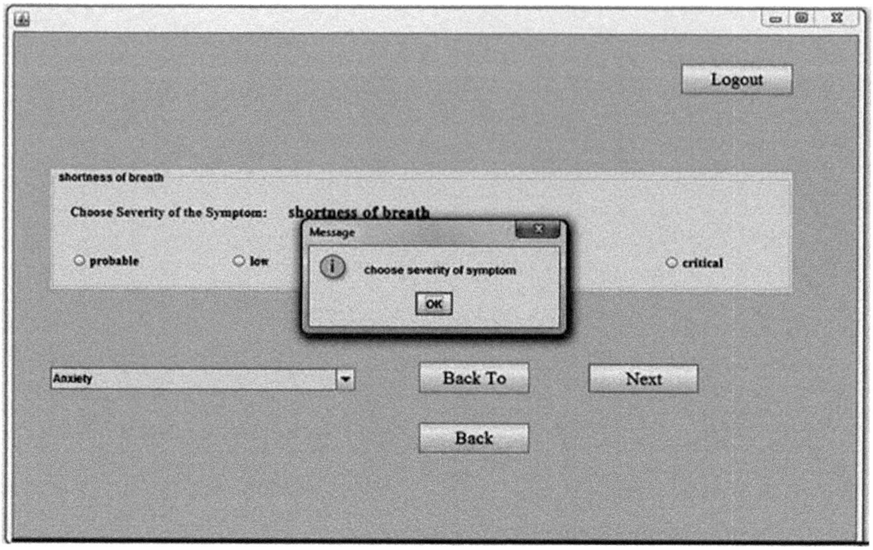

FIGURE 6.17 (*Continued*) (a) Choosing severity of the symptom. (b) Choosing severity of the symptom.

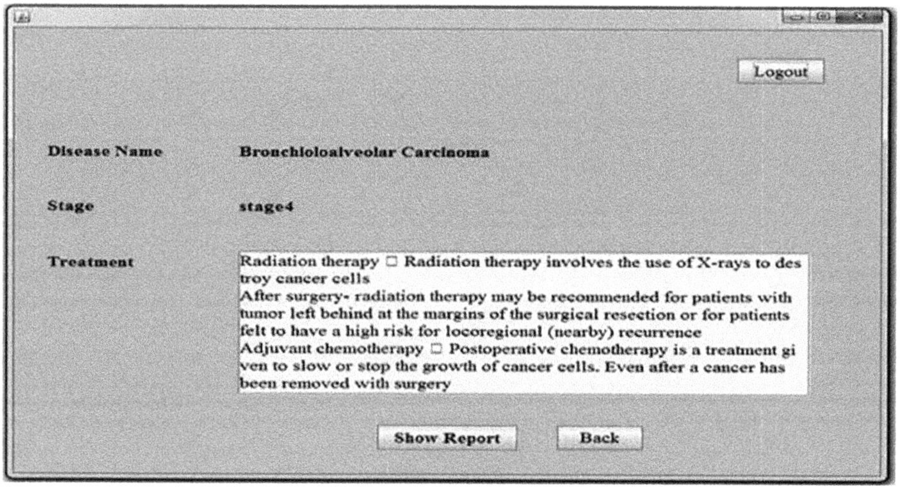

FIGURE 6.18 Displaying disease name along with stage.

- View Number of Users
- View User Reports
- Add New Diseases
- Update Treatment

The user can select one to proceed further.

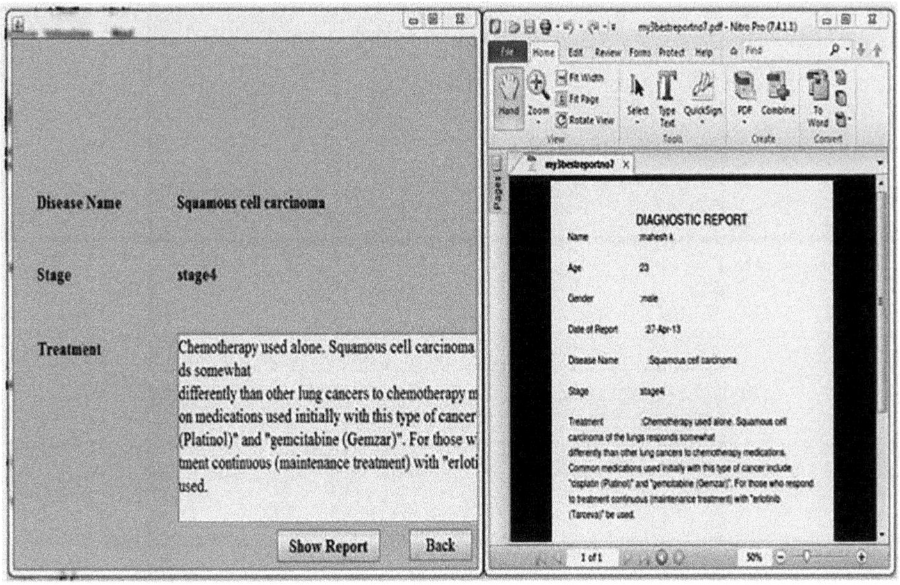

FIGURE 6.19 Diagnostic report of the patient.

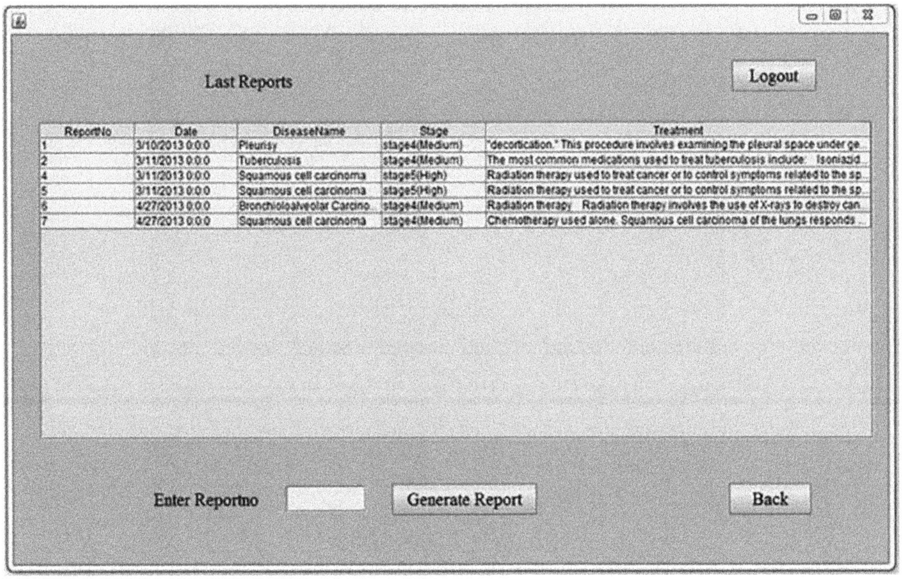

FIGURE 6.20 Displaying the last reports.

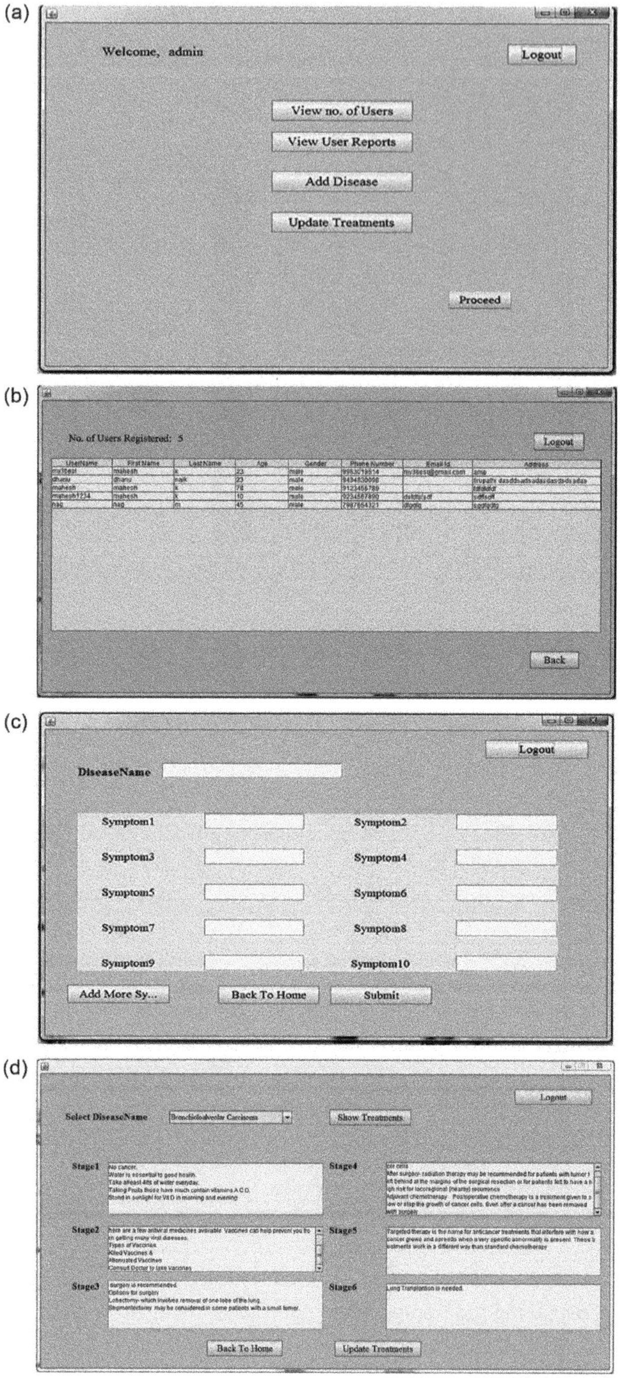

FIGURE 6.21 (a) Expert panel screen. (b) No of users. (c) Add new disease name. (d) Update treatment.

6.7 CONCLUSIONS

This Novel Predictive system has evolved as an Internet-based standalone application, and it can be used by both patients as well as doctors. The systems validation is conducted by comparing the system-generated outputs with doctor annotations. It is found that the results generated by the system are 85% accurate. The system can be extended to handle imagery data and numerical data. The knowledge base may be enhanced by incorporating machine learning capabilities into the existing system. Datasets may be collected from various geographically different areas and incorporated into the system design so that personalized recommendation systems may be provided to the users.

REFERENCES

1. A. Hashemi, A. H. Pilevar, R. Rafeh, "Mass Detection in Lung CT Images Using Region Growing Segmentation and Decision Making Based on Fuzzy Inference System and Artificial Neural Network," *International Journal of Image, Graphics, and Signal Processing*, Vol. 5, No. 6, pp. 16–24, 2013.
2. S. Sivakumar, Dr. C. Chandrasekar, "Lung Nodule Detection Using Fuzzy Clustering and Support Vector Machines," *International Journal of Engineering and Technology (IJET)*, Vol. 5, No. 1, pp. 179–185, Feb-Mar 2013.
3. R. K. Ada, "Early Detection and Prediction of Lung Cancer Survival Using Neural Network Classifier," *International Journal of Application or Innovation in Engineering and Management*, Vol. 2, No. 6, pp. 375–383, June 2013. ISSN: 2319-4847.
4. Dr. D. P. Shukla, S. B. Patel, A. K. Sen, "A Literature Review in Health Informatics the Use of Data Mining Techniques," *International Journal of Software and Hardware Research in Engineering*, Vol. 2, , pp. 123–129, Feb 2014. ISSN: 2347-4890.
5. B. Venkatalakshmi, M. V. Shivsankar, "Heart Disease Diagnosis Using Predictive Data Mining," *International Journal of Innovative Research in Science, Engineering and Technology*, Vol. 3, pp. 1873–1877, Mar. 2014.
6. R. Hermon, P. A. H. Williams, "Big Data in Healthcare: What Is It Used for?" *Proceedings of the 3rd Australian e-Health Informatics and Security Conference*, Edith, 1–3 December 2014, DOI:10.4225/75/57982b9431b48.
7. R. M. Luque-Baena, D. Urda, M. G. Claros, L. Franco, J. M. Jerez, "Robust Gene Signatures from Microarray Data Using Genetic Algorithms Enriched with Biological Pathway Keywords," *Journal of Biomedical Informatics*, Vol. 49, pp. 32–44, 2014.
8. A. S. Moussa, S. A. Yones, "Tumor Volume Fuzzification for Intelligent Cancer Staging," *Applied Soft Computing*, Vol. 35, pp. 227–236, October 2015.
9. P. Nithya, B. Umamaheshwari, R. Deepa, "Detection of Lung Cancer Using Data Mining Classification Techniques," *International Journal of Advanced Research in Computer Science and Software Engineering*, Vol. 5, No. 7, pp. 1060–1062, July 2015.
10. L. Qin, V. Atluri. "Concept-Level Access Control for the Semantic Web," In *Proceedings of the 2003 ACM Workshop on XML Security - XMLSEC 03* (pp. 94–103)2003.
11. "Ontology Development and Optimization for Data Integration and Decision-Making in Product Design and Obsolescence Management," *Ontology Modeling in Physical Asset Integrity Management*, 87–132, 2015.
12. K. Senthamaraikannan, N. SenthilvelMurugan, V. Vallinayagam, T. Viveka, "Analysis of Liver Cancer DNA Sequence Data Using Data Mining," *International Journal of Computer Applications (0975–8887)*, Vol. 61, No. 3, pp. 23–25, January 2013.

13. E. Magdy, N. Zayed, M. Fakhr, "Automatic Classification of Normal and Cancer Lung CT Images Using Multiscale AM-FM Features," *International Journal of Biomedical Imaging*, Vol. 2015, 7 p, 2015. Article ID 230830.
14. S. Vijayarani, S. Sudha, "An Efficient Clustering Algorithm for Predicting Diseases from Hemogram Blood Test Samples," *Indian Journal of Science and Technology*, Vol. 8, pp. 1–8, Aug. 2015.
15. B. Al-Hamadani, T. Shubita, "Novel Hyper-Active Algorithm to Estimate Missing Microarray Attributes," *Computer and Information Science*, Vol. 8, No. 3, p. 10, 2015.
16. Computer Science & Information Technology (CS & IT), https://www.airccj.org/CSCP/vol6/csit65201.pdf, pp. 01–09, 2016. © CS & IT-CSCP 2016. DOI:10.5121/csit.2016.60501.
17. J. Thomas, R. T. Princy, "Human Heart Disease Prediction System Using Data Mining Techniques," *2016 International Conference on Circuit, Power and Computing Technologies (ICCPCT)*. IEEE, 4 Aug 2016. DOI:10.1109/ICCPCT.2016.7530265.
18. V. Krishnaiah, Dr. G. Narsimha, N. Subhash Chandra, "Diagnosis of Lung Cancer Prediction System Using Data Mining Classification Techniques," *(IJCSIT) International Journal of Computer Science and Information Technologies*, Vol. 4, No. 1, pp. 39–45, 2013.
19. *International Journal of Science and Research (IJSR)*. ISSN (Online): 2319–7064 Index Copernicus Value (2013): 6.14 | Impact Factor (2013): 4.438.
20. K. A. Ahmed, S. Aljahdali, S. N. Hussain, "Comparative Prediction Performance with Support Vector Machine and Random Forest Classification Techniques," *International Journal of Computer Applications*, Vol. 69, No. 11, pp. 12–16, 2013.
21. R. Chitra, V. Seenivasagam, "Review of Heart Disease Prediction System Using Data Mining and Hybrid Intelligent Techniques," *ICTACT Journal on Soft Computing*, Vol. 3, pp. 605–609, July 2013.
22. R. Ozcan, Y. A. Aslandogan, "Concept Based Information Retrieval Using Ontologies and Latent Semantic Analysis," A Technical Report, CSE-2004-8, 2004.
23. M. Lichman, *UCI Machine Learning Repository*. https://archive.ics.uci.edu/ml. Irvine, CA: The University of California, School of Information and Computer Science, 2013.
24. Ahmad, A., F. Miad, "Augmenting Breath Regulation Using a Mobile Driven Virtual Reality Therapy Framework," *IEEE Journal of Biomedical and Health Informatics*, Vol. 18, No. 3, pp. 746–752, 2013.
25. www.rajpub.com
26. Ebrahimipour, V., & Yacout, S. (Eds.). *Ontology Modeling in Physical Asset Integrity Management*. Cham: Springer International Publishing, 2015.
27. Mr. Vijay A. Gajdhane, Professor L. M. Deshpande, "Detection of Lung Cancer Stages on CT Scan Images by Using Various Image Processing Techniques," *IOSR Journal of Computer Engineering*, Vol. 16, No. 5, pp. 28–35, Sep–Oct 2014.
28. S. A. Yones, A. S. Moussa, H. Hassan, N. H. Alieldin, "On the Significance of Fuzzification of the N and M in Cancer Staging," *Cancer Informatics*, Vol. 13, pp. 85–91, March 2014.
29. S. K. Saini, Gaurav, A. Choudhary, "Detection of Lung Carcinoma Using Fuzzy Logic and ACO Techniques," *International Journal of Engineering Research & Technology (IJERT)*, Vol. 3, No. 8, pp. 903–906, 2014.
30. Mr.Vijay A. Gajdhane, Prof. L. M. Deshpande, "Detection of Lung Cancer Nodule on Computed Tomography Images by Using Image Processing," *International Journal of Application or Innovation in Engineering & Management (IJAIEM)*, Vol. 3, No. 7, 281–285, July 2014.

7 Identification of Brain Tumors in MRI Images Using Artificial Intelligence of Things

Ganesh Khekare, Goutam Majumder, Ganesh Yenurkar, Gopal Sakarkar, Urvashi Dhanre, and Bhushan Vidhale

7.1 INTRODUCTION

The use of Artificial Intelligence of Things in medical imaging has improved diagnostic accuracy and facilitated the early detection of diseases, particularly in the context of tumor detection. Magnetic resonance imaging (MRI) is a frequently used health imaging procedure known for its ability to provide detailed anatomical information. However, the interpretation of MRI images can be challenging and time-consuming for medical professionals, especially when identifying subtle tumor structures [1].

The important contribution of this research work is to explore and implement different Machine Learning algorithms and approaches to develop an efficient and accurate tumor detection system for MRI images. This research aimed to address the following objectives:

- **Literature review**: Conducting an in-depth review of existing research papers, publications, and state-of-the-art methods in the area of Machine Learning for health data analysis and tumor detection in MRI.
- **Data preparation**: Acquiring and preprocessing MRI datasets containing labeled tumor images and normal tissues, ensuring data quality and consistency for training and evaluation.
- **Architecture selection**: Evaluating different Deep Learning architectures, such as ResNet, DenseNet, VGG19, VGG16, and custom-designed Convolutional Neural Network layers, to determine the most suitable models for tumor detection tasks.
- **Feature extraction**: Investigating various feature extraction methods to represent MRI images effectively, capturing relevant information for tumor identification [2].

DOI: 10.1201/9781003469896-7

- **Model training**: Training the selected Machine Learning models using the preprocessed MRI dataset to learn patterns and correlations between tumor regions and normal tissues.
- **Performance evaluation**: Assessing the performance of the trained models using metrics such as accuracy.
- **Interpretability and visualization**: Exploring techniques for model interpretability and visualizing the decision-making process to gain insights into the learned features and enhance the trustworthiness of the system [3].

The successful development of an accurate and reliable tumor detection system can significantly assist medical professionals in diagnosing and treating patients more effectively [4]. The area of health imaging faces the critical challenge of timely and accurate identification of disease using magnetic resonance imaging (MRI) pictures. The prediction of these data is critical and time-consuming, often leading to delays in diagnosis and treatment planning. Conventional manual analysis by medical professionals may also result in subjective assessments and potential errors [5]. To address these issues, this research project aimed to harness the power of Artificial Intelligence of Things to develop an effective and reliable disease detection and classification system. The primary problem at hand is to design and implement machine learning models capable of accurately distinguishing between normal brain images and those containing tumors. Furthermore, the research aimed to extend this capability to differentiate various types of brain tumors, enhancing the diagnostic process by providing insights into tumor characteristics. The complex nature of MRI images, coupled with the diversity of tumor shapes, sizes, and locations, presents a multifaceted problem. Developing models capable of capturing these intricate patterns and enabling rapid, non-invasive diagnosis requires a comprehensive exploration of various machine learning algorithms, advanced preprocessing techniques, and the integration of domain-specific knowledge [6].

The goal of this research work was to contribute to the improvement of medical diagnosis and patient care by creating a robust and interpretable brain tumor detection and classification system. The project sought to address the limitations of manual analysis and offer medical professionals a tool that can aid in early detection, accurate classification, and informed decision-making. By aligning the project with this problem definition, the research aimed to bridge the gap between cutting-edge Artificial Intelligence of Things and the pressing need for efficient brain tumor analysis, potentially revolutionizing medical imaging practices and patient outcomes. The rest of the chapter is bifurcated as Section 7.2 provides a literature review, Section 7.3 describes the methodology used, Section 7.4 describes the implementation and result discussion, and Section 7.5 is the conclusion followed by references used. The chapter concludes by discussing future avenues for enhancing the project's outcomes, including more advanced preprocessing techniques, ensembling methods, and exploration of rare tumor types.

7.2 LITERATURE REVIEW

The paper by Ankit Ghosh and Alok Kole presents [7,8] a comprehensive empirical analysis of machine-learning algorithms for brain tumor identification. The authors explore the application of nine different ML algorithms, including Support Vector Machine [9,10], Random Forest, Logistic Regression, Gradient, Naïve Bayes, K means, Decision Tree, LSTM, XGBoost, etc. on data consisting of MRI brain pictures [11,12]. The study evaluates the performance of these algorithms based on various parameters, like accuracy, recollect, exactitude, F1-Score, AUC-ROC slopes, and AUC-PR slopes. After rigorous iterations, the results indicate that Gradient Boosting provides better results of classification as compared to other Machine Learning classifiers tested [10,13]. Additionally, the authors implemented multi-level classification on various datasets consisting of brain MRI pictures of glioma, meningioma, pituitary, and non-tumor using Support Vector Machine, Random Forest, K Nearest Neighbor, and XG Boost classifiers [14,15]. The XGBoost classifier demonstrated superior performance, outperforming the other classifiers in accuracy, recall, precision, F1-score, and AUC-ROC score [16,17]. Brain tumor detection in the early stage is still the biggest challenge faced by doctors.

In summary, the research paper "A Comparative Study of Enhanced Machine Learning Algorithms for Brain Tumor Detection and Classification" explores the use of ML classification techniques for disease analysis from MRI pictures [18,19]. The authors propose a hybrid method integrating Convolutional Neural Networks (CNN) and Support Vector Machines (SVM) to gain high accuracy in classification [20]. The results demonstrate that the hybrid CNN-SVM model outperforms individual SVM and CNN models in terms of accuracy. As a result of this study, the focus has shifted towards using deep learning methods [21,22], particularly CNN-SVM hybrid models, due to their superior performance in achieving higher accuracy metrics in brain tumor classification [23].

The article presents a hybrid approach using a Convolutional Neural Network (CNN) and Support Vector Machine (SVM) for tumor analysis of the MRI brain dataset. The proposed system outperforms traditional machine learning methods [24] and shows significant improvements in accuracy [25]. The combination of CNN [26] and SVM allows for better feature reuse and gradient flow, leading to enhanced model compactness and performance. The study emphasizes the importance of non-invasive, computer-aided diagnosis tools in handling brain tumors and improving diagnostic accuracy within seconds. Though lots of techniques are already available the system which predicts accurately is still missing. A strong, robust system is needed which predicts the brain tumor promptly.

7.3 METHODOLOGY

This research focused on the analysis of brain MRI image datasets using artificial intelligence (AI) methods, specifically for tumor detection and classification. Two datasets were utilized in the study. The first dataset involved binary classification to distinguish between healthy brain images and those with tumors. The second dataset comprised multi-class classification to analyze various types of brain tumors. Throughout the research, a series of well-defined stages are executed, including dataset preparation, model construction, training and evaluation, performance comparison, and result analysis. Initial efforts involved the development of a custom three-layer convolutional neural network (CNN) that demonstrated impressive accuracy in binary classification. CNNs have emerged as powerful tools for facial emotion recognition due to their ability to automatically learn discriminative features from raw pixel data. By leveraging deep learning techniques, CNNs can achieve high accuracy in emotion classification tasks. Subsequently, pre-trained systems such as DenseNet, ResNet, VGG16, and VGG19 are employed for tumor-type classification.

The primary tasks in this research include:

1. **Dataset preparation**: The brain MRI image datasets were collected from online sources, specifically from Kaggle. The datasets were preprocessed to ensure uniformity and eliminate any inconsistencies in the images. The preprocessing steps involved resizing, normalization, and noise reduction.
2. **Model construction**: Several machine learning and deep learning systems were developed for the tasks of tumor detection and classification. Commonly used models such as Support Vector Machine (SVM), Convolutional Neural Network (CNN), and others were considered.
3. **Training and evaluation**: The prepared datasets were bifurcated into training and testing datasets. The systems were trained on the training dataset using appropriate optimization techniques. The trained models were then evaluated on the testing data to assess their performance.
4. **Performance comparison**: The models' performances were compared based on various evaluation metrics, with accuracy being the primary metric of interest. The model with the appropriate accuracy was identified as the best-performing system.
5. **Result analysis**: The final step involved analyzing the results of the models and interpreting their predictions. The insights gained from the analysis were used to conclude the accuracy of different AI algorithms in brain tumor detection and classification tasks.

Throughout the project, the focus was on leveraging advanced AI techniques to handle medical image datasets, particularly MRI brain images. The aim was to develop accurate and efficient models that can aid in the quick identification and classification of brain tumors, contributing to improved medical diagnosis and treatment planning.

7.4 IMPLEMENTATION AND RESULT DISCUSSION

7.4.1 Work Stages

- **Literature review and methodology exploration**: Conducted a comprehensive review of relevant research papers and methodologies used in brain tumor detection and classification. Explored online courses, documentation of applied libraries, and machine learning methods.

- **Dataset identification and preparation**: Identified suitable brain MRI image datasets for the project's objectives. Prepared the datasets by ensuring uniformity and preprocessing steps like resizing normalization, and noise reduction, as output these kinds of pictures with labels as shown in Figures 7.1 and 7.2.
- **Initial model building and training**: Started building preliminary models for binary classification (healthy vs. tumor) using the prepared dataset as shown in Figure 7.3. Trained these models and analyzed their performance.

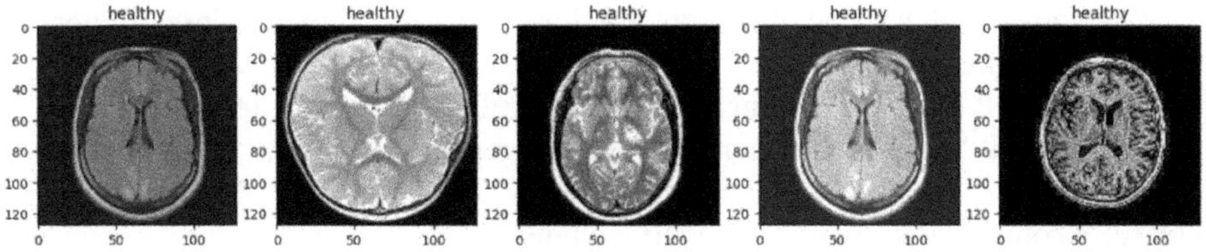

FIGURE 7.1 Pictures with no tumor.

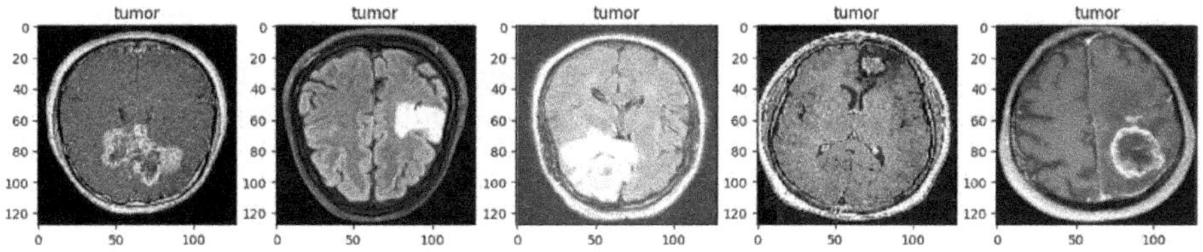

FIGURE 7.2 Pictures a tumor.

```
CNN(
  (cnn_model): Sequential(
    (0): Conv2d(3, 6, kernel_size=(5, 5), stride=(1, 1))
    (1): Tanh()
    (2): AvgPool2d(kernel_size=2, stride=5, padding=0)
    (3): Conv2d(6, 16, kernel_size=(5, 5), stride=(1, 1))
    (4): Tanh()
    (5): AvgPool2d(kernel_size=2, stride=5, padding=0)
  )
  (fc_model): Sequential(
    (0): Linear(in_features=256, out_features=120, bias=True)
    (1): Tanh()
    (2): Linear(in_features=120, out_features=84, bias=True)
    (3): Tanh()
    (4): Linear(in_features=84, out_features=1, bias=True)
  )
)
```

FIGURE 7.3 The architecture of the constructed neural network.

The network consists of two main parts: a convolutional section (cnn_model) and a fully connected section (fc_model).

The convolutional section (cnn_model) includes:

- **Convolutional layer (Conv2d)**: Applies a 5×5 convolutional kernel to the input image, generating 6 feature maps that represent different learned features.
- **Tanh activation (Tanh)**: Apply the hyperbolic tangent activation function to introduce non-linearity after each convolutional layer.
- **Average Pooling layer (AvgPool2d)**: Performs average pooling over 2×2 windows with a stride of 5, reducing dimensionality while retaining important features.
- **Repeats 2 and 3 for the next convolutional layer**: Similar to the first convolutional layer, another convolution, activation, and pooling are applied.

The fully connected section (fc_model) includes:

- **Fully connected layer (linear)**: Transforms the data from the last convolutional layer into a vector and passes it through a fully connected layer. It has 256 input features and 120 output features.
- **Tanh activation**: Applies the hyperbolic tangent activation function again.
- **Fully connected layer**: Takes the 120 input features and compresses them into 84 output features.
- **Tanh activation**: Applies the hyperbolic tangent activation function once more.
- **Fully connected layer**: The final layer of the fully connected section has 1 output feature, which could indicate a binary classification or regression decision.

This CNN architecture extracts features from input images and makes decisions based on the specific task it's designed for. For MRI images in our case.

Let's consider one image as shown in Figure 7.4.

As it goes through the network - certain features stand out to send it to a fully connected layer.

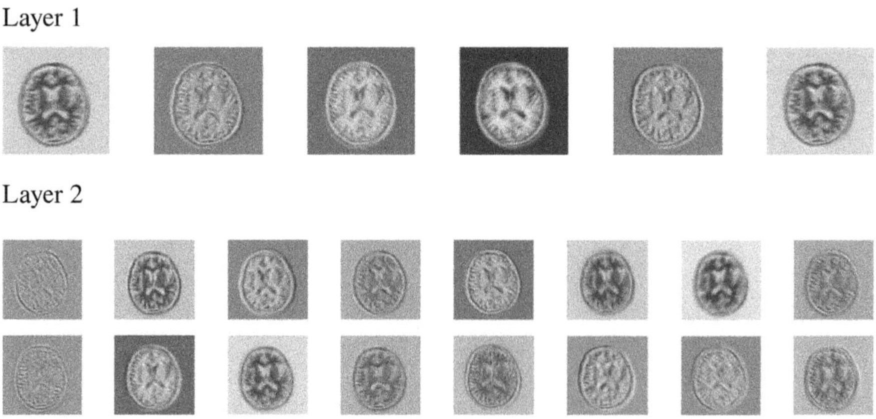

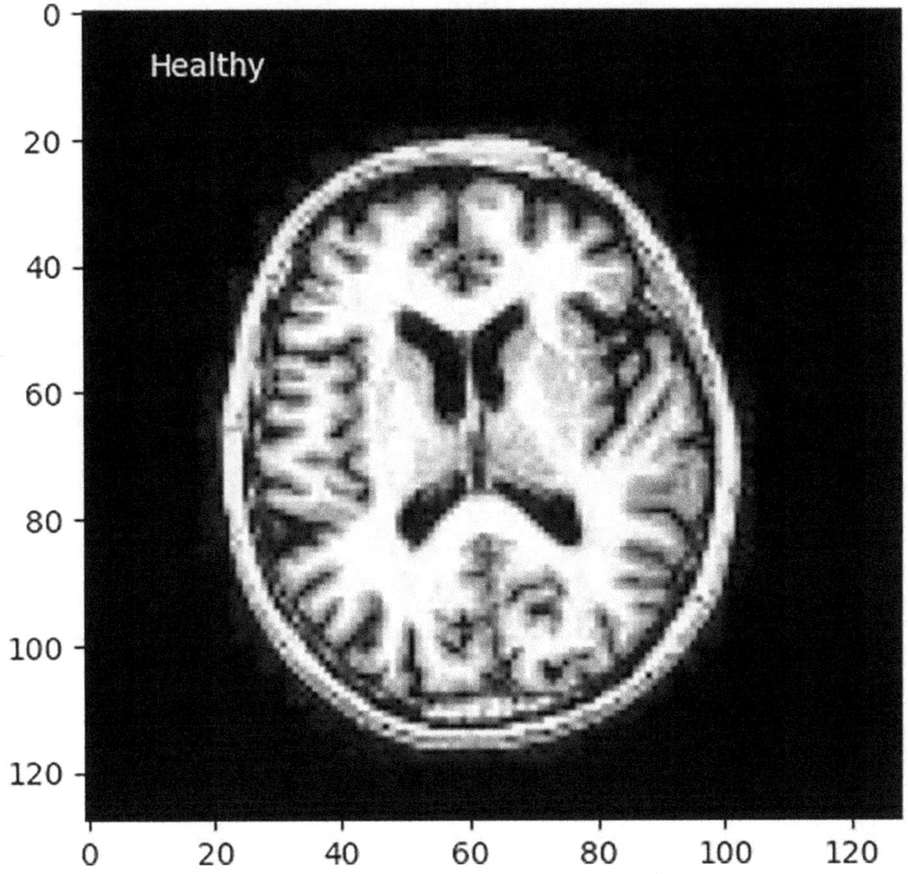

FIGURE 7.4 Random image from the dataset.

And that is sent to the fully connected layer. After training, the results are:

- **Test accuracy**: 0.940000 Through this graph, it can be mentioned that the model has learned training samples on the 150th epoch, as shown in Figure 7.5.
- **Dataset selection for multi-class classification**: Selecting a dataset for the differentiation of various types of diseases.
- **Data preparation for multi-class classification**: Prepared the data for multi-class classification, ensuring it meets the requirements of the chosen models.
- **Pretrained model exploration and training**: Explored pre-trained models suitable for image analysis and utilized them for transfer learning. Trained these models on the selected dataset for brain tumor classification. Multiple training sessions were conducted due to the time-intensive nature of training each model.
- **Results comparison and analysis**: Compare the results of different models and evaluate their performance based on various metrics like accuracy.

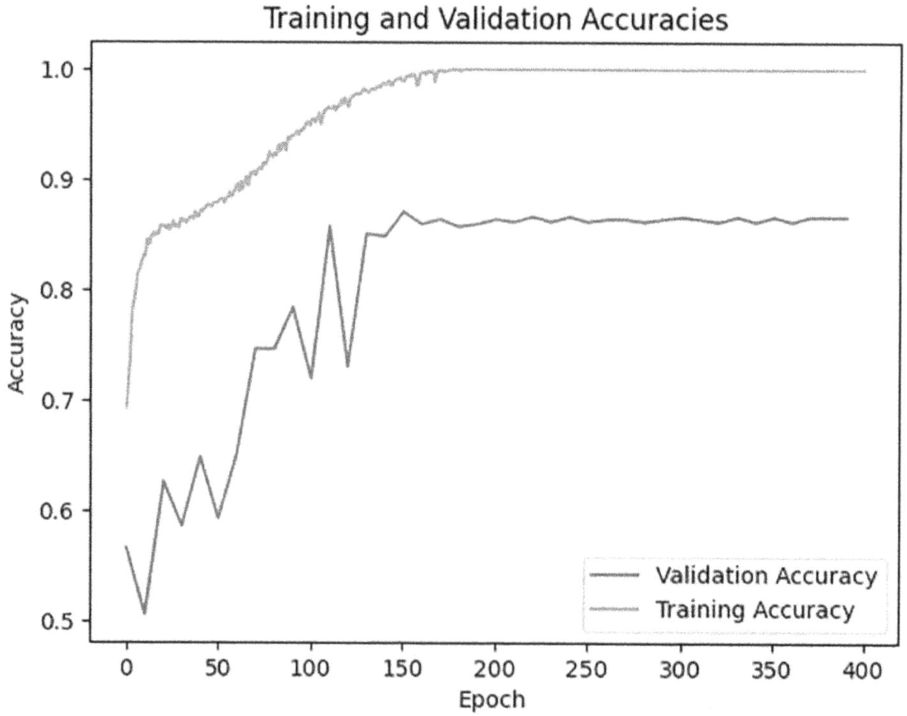

FIGURE 7.5 Validation and training accuracy.

Several graphs for accuracy on different models are shown in Figure 7.6.

Each model was trained for more than two hours. Throughout this research work, a significant portion of my time was dedicated to understanding the practical aspects of using existing tools and libraries for creating and training models. Learning how to work with pre-trained systems and fine-tuning them for specific tasks was particularly time-consuming. This work allowed for a comprehensive exploration of brain tumor identification using AI techniques and provided valuable insights into medical image analysis applications.

The initial custom-built three-layer convolutional neural network (CNN) with a simple architecture and fully connected layers demonstrated a remarkable test accuracy of 0.94 for the binary classification task, effectively distinguishing between healthy brain images and those with tumors. Subsequently, they employed pre-trained systems, namely DenseNet, ResNet, VGG16, and VGG19, to tackle the binary classification task. While these models exhibited only slight improvements in accuracy compared to the custom CNN, they showcased their true potential when confronted with the more challenging task of tumor type classification.

For the tumor type classification task, DenseNet achieved an accuracy of 0.8889, ResNet achieved an accuracy of 0.8720, VGG16 achieved an accuracy of 0.8575, and VGG19 achieved an accuracy of 0.8442. These models outperformed the custom CNN and showcased their ability to accurately classify brain tumor types into three categories: glioma, meningioma, and pituitary. The confusion matrixes revealed the models' capability to distinguish between the different tumor types, effectively

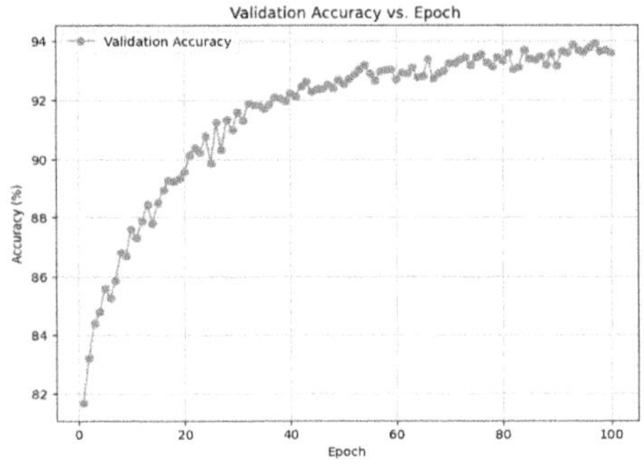

DenseNet

Accuracy on test data: 0.8889

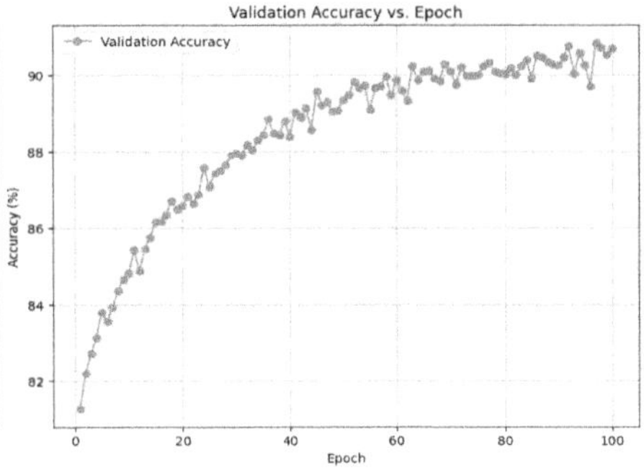

ResNet

Accuracy on test data: 0.8720

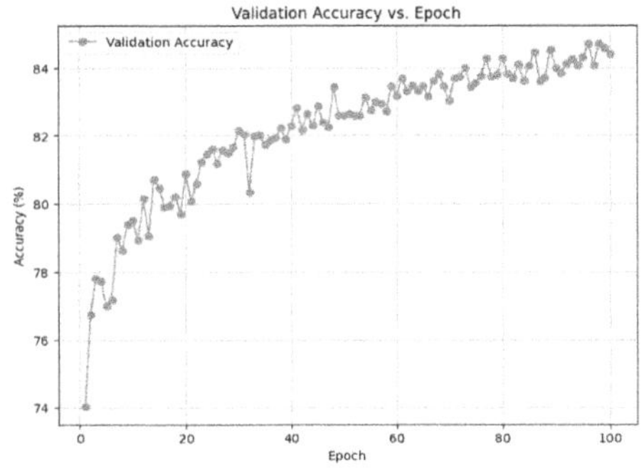

VGG16

Accuracy on test data: 0.8575

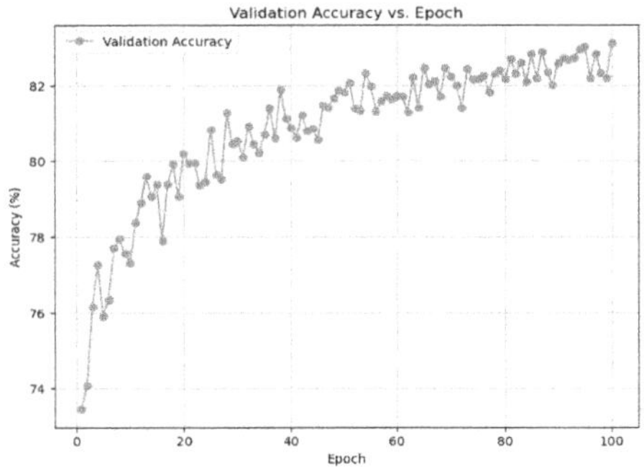

VGG19

Accuracy on test data: 0.8442

FIGURE 7.6 Comparative evaluation of model accuracy.

contributing to medical diagnosis and treatment planning. Overall, the results highlight the superiority of pre-trained models for complex classification tasks involving brain tumor imaging datasets. The use of these models provides valuable insights into tumor classification, thereby increasing the perfection of the system. This research work significantly contributed to the development and implementation of powerful machine-learning models for brain tumor classification using MRI images. The achieved results demonstrate the potential of AI-based approaches in assisting medical professionals in accurate diagnosis and improved treatment decisions for brain tumor patients. The experience of exploring and utilizing pre-trained systems, such as DenseNet, ResNet, VGG16, and VGG19, not only expanded knowledge but also demonstrated the versatility and power of transfer learning in health data analysis. This research work has deepened my appreciation for the importance of domain-specific knowledge, data preprocessing, and the interpretability of model results in the medical domain. Moreover, extending the classification to include more rare tumor types and exploring the potential for transfer learning from other medical imaging domains could yield valuable insights and contribute to the advancement of medical research.

7.5 CONCLUSION

Significant progress was achieved through this research in brain tumor classification using magnetic resonance imaging (MRI) datasets. Initially, a custom-built three-layer CNN was developed, which demonstrated high accuracy in binary classification, effectively distinguishing between healthy brain images and those with tumors. The work was carried out via the Python language and the Pytorch libraries for working with deep learning. Further exploration involved using pre-trained systems, including DenseNet, ResNet, VGG16, and VGG19, for the more challenging task of tumor type classification. The pre-trained models exhibited improved performance compared to the custom CNN, perfectly bifurcating brain tumor types into three parts: glioma, meningioma, and pituitary. The successful implementation of these models enables effective medical diagnosis and treatment planning by providing valuable insights into tumor classification based on MRI images. The results obtained are promising and underscore the potential for using advanced Artificial Intelligence of Things in the medical imaging domain. While substantial progress was made during this research work, there are still areas for further improvement and exploration. One aspect that could be explored is the incorporation of more advanced pre-processing techniques to improve the validity of input data. The application of ensembling methods and other deep learning architectures might lead to further performance improvements.

This research work provided an invaluable opportunity to immerse one in the world of machine learning, necessitating a significant amount of time devoted to learning and understanding the practical application of various methods. Working on the project allowed people to gain hands-on experience handling real-world datasets, preprocessing image data, selecting appropriate models, and tuning hyperparameters for optimal performance. The process of implementing and training different models, as well as analyzing their results, enhanced the understanding of the intricacies and challenges involved in applying Artificial Intelligence of Things to the medical field.

REFERENCES

1. M. Rasool, N. A. Ismail, W. Boulila, A. Ammar, H. Samma, W. M. S. Yafooz, and A. M. Emara, "A Hybrid Deep Learning Model for Brain Tumour Classification," *Entropy (Basel)*, vol. 24, no. 6, p. 799, June 8, 2022. DOI: 10.3390/e24060799.
2. (a) M. O. Khairandish, M. Sharma, V. Jain, J. M. Chatterjee, and N. Z. Jhanjhi, "A Hybrid CNN-SVM Threshold Segmentation Approach for Tumor Detection and Classification of MRI Brain Images," *IRBM*, vol. 42, no. 5, pp. 307–316, 2021. (b) B. Raghuram, and B. Hanumanthu, "Brain Tumor Image Identification and Classification on the Internet of Medical Things Using Deep Learning," *Measurement: Sensors*, vol. 30, p. 100905, 2023. ISSN 2665-9174. DOI: 10.1016/j.measen.2023.100905. (https://www.sciencedirect.com/science/article/pii/S2665917423002416)
3. M. Z. Khaliki, and M. S. Başarslan, "Brain Tumor Detection from Images and Comparison with Transfer Learning Methods and 3-Layer CNN," *Scienctific Reports*, vol. 14, p. 2664, 2024. DOI: 10.1038/s41598-024-52823-9.

4. A. Ghosh, and A. Kole, "A Comparative Study of Enhanced Machine Learning Algorithms for Brain Tumor Detection and Classification," *TechRxiv*, Institute of Electrical and Electronics Engineers (IEEE), 2021.
5. G. Khekare, and P. Verma, "Prophetic Probe of Accidents in Indian Smart Cities Using Machine Learning." In: Bhateja, V., Satapathy, S. C., Travieso-González, C. M., Aradhya, V. N. M. (eds), *Data Engineering and Intelligent Computing. Advances in Intelligent Systems and Computing*, vol 1407. Springer, Singapore, 2021. DOI: 10.1007/978-981-16-0171-2_18.
6. J. S. Suri, and Y. Chitre, "Multiclass Magnetic Resonance Imaging Brain Tumor Classification Using Artificial Intelligence Paradigm," *Computers in Biology and Medicine*, vol. 122, p. 103804, 2020.
7. Z. Jia, and D. Chen, "Brain Tumor Identification and Classification of MRI Images Using Deep Learning Techniques," *IEEE Access*. DOI: 10.1109/ACCESS.2020.3016319.
8. G. Khekare, and K. Solanki, "Real Time Object Detection with Speech Recognition Using Tensorflow Lite," *GIS Science Journal*, vol. 9, no. 3, p. 552, 2022.
9. B. Deepa, M. Murugappan, M. G. Sumithra, M. Mahmud, and M. S. Al-Rakhami, "Pattern Descriptors Orientation and MAP Firefly Algorithm Based Brain Pathology Classification Using Hybridized Machine Learning Algorithm," *IEEE Access*, vol. 10, pp. 3848–3863, 2022. DOI: 10.1109/ACCESS.2021.3100549.
10. Y. Ma, Q. Wang, L. Cao, L. Li, C. Zhang, L. Qiao, and M. Liu, "Multi-Scale Dynamic Graph Learning for Brain Disorder Detection With Functional MRI," *IEEE Transactions on Neural Systems and Rehabilitation Engineering*, vol. 31, pp. 3501–3512, 2023. DOI: 10.1109/TNSRE.2023.3309847.
11. G. Khekare, Y. Patel, P. Nishit, D. Engineer, and P. Badal, "Detection of Brain Tumor Using Data Science: A Survey," *International Journal of Engineering Applied Sciences and Technology*, vol. 6, no. 9, pp. 2455–2143, 2022.
12. N. Saeed, M. Ridzuan, H. Alasmawi, I. Sobirov, and M. Yaqub, "MGMT Promoter Methylation Status Prediction Using MRI Scans? An Extensive Experimental Evaluation of Deep Learning Models," *Medical Image Analysis*, vol. 90, p. 102989, 2023. ISSN 1361-8415. DOI: 10.1016/j.media.2023.102989.
13. T. A. Soomro, L. Zheng, A. J. Afifi, A. Ali, S. Soomro, M. Yin, and J. Gao, "Image Segmentation for MR Brain Tumor Detection Using Machine Learning: A Review," *IEEE Reviews in Biomedical Engineering*, vol. 16, pp. 70–90, 2023. DOI: 10.1109/RBME.2022.3185292.
14. Z. Atha, and J. Chaki, "SSBTCNet: Semi-Supervised Brain Tumor Classification Network," *IEEE Access*, vol. 11, pp. 141485–141499, 2023. DOI: 10.1109/ACCESS.2023.3343126.
15. B. Mallampati, A. Ishaq, F. Rustam, V. Kuthala, S. Alfarhood, and I. Ashraf, "Brain Tumor Detection Using 3D-UNet Segmentation Features and Hybrid Machine Learning Model," *IEEE Access*, vol. 11, pp. 135020–135034, 2023. DOI: 10.1109/ACCESS.2023.3337363.
16. D. S. Vinod, S. P. S. Prakash, H. AlSalman, A. Y. Muaad, and M. B. B. Heyat, "Ensemble Technique for Brain Tumor Patient Survival Prediction," *IEEE Access*, vol. 12, pp. 19285–19298, 2024. DOI: 10.1109/ACCESS.2024.3360086.
17. B. Sandhiya, and S. K. S. Raja, "Deep Learning and Optimized Learning Machine for Brain Tumor Classification," *Biomedical Signal Processing and Control*, vol. 89, p. 105778, 2024. ISSN: 1746-8094. DOI: 10.1016/j.bspc.2023.105778.
18. S. Anantharajan, S. Gunasekaran, T. Subramanian, and R. Venkatesh, "MRI Brain Tumor Detection Using Deep Learning and Machine Learning Approaches," *Measurement: Sensors*, vol. 31, p. 101026, 2024. ISSN 2665-9174. DOI: 10.1016/j.measen.2024.101026.

19. H. Hwang, S. E. Kim, H. -J. Lee, D. A. Lee, and K. M. Park, "Identification of Amnestic Mild Cognitive Impairment by Structural and Functional MRI Using a Machine-Learning Approach," *Clinical Neurology and Neurosurgery*, p. 108177, 2024. ISSN 0303-8467. DOI: 10.1016/j.clineuro.2024.108177.
20. G. Khekare, K. Pavan Kumar, K. N. Prasanthi, S. R. Godla, V. Rachapudi, M. S. Al Ansari, and Y. A. Baker El-Ebiary, "Optimizing Network Security and Performance through the Integration of Hybrid GAN-RNN Models in SDN-Based Access Control and Traffic Engineering," *International Journal of Advanced Computer Science and Applications (IJACSA)*, vol. 14, no. 12, 2023. DOI: 10.14569/IJACSA.2023.0141262.
21. G. Khekare, and Midhunchakkravarthy, "Smart Image Recognition System for the Visually Impaired People." In: *2023 International Conference on Energy, Materials and Communication Engineering (ICEMCE)*, Madurai, India, 2023, pp. 1–6. DOI: 10.1109/ICEMCE57940.2023.10434130.
22. A. V. N. Reddy, P. K. Mallick, B. Srinivasa Rao, and P. Kanakamedala, "An Efficient Brain Tumor Classification Using MRI Images with Hybrid Deep Intelligence Model," *The Imaging Science Journal*, 2023. DOI: 10.1080/13682199.2023.2207892.
23. S. Aluri, and S. S. Imambi "Brain Tumour Classification Using MRI Images Based on Lenet with Golden Teacher Learning Optimization," *Network: Computation in Neural Systems*, vol. 35, no. 1, pp. 27–54, 2024. DOI: 10.1080/0954898X.2023.2275720.
24. M. Kordemir, K. K. Cevik, and A. Bozkurt, "A Mask R-CNN Approach for Detection and Classification of Brain Tumours from MR Images," *Computer Methods in Biomechanics and Biomedical Engineering: Imaging & Visualization,* 2024. DOI: 10.1080/21681163.2023.2301391.
25. S. Raju, and V. R. Peddireddy Veera, "Classification of Brain Tumours from MRI Images Using Deep Learning-Enabled Hybrid Optimization Algorithm," *Network: Computation in Neural Systems*, vol. 34, no. 4, pp. 408–437, 2023. DOI: 10.1080/0954898X.2023.2275045.
26. R. D. Chougala, and R. H. Havaldar, "Systematic Assessment and Review of Techniques Based on Tumour Detection in Brain Using MRI," *Computer Methods in Biomechanics and Biomedical Engineering: Imaging & Visualization*, vol. 11, no. 5, pp. 1708–1716, 2023. DOI: 10.1080/21681163.2023.2181020.

8 Transformative Insights

Image-Based Breast Cancer Detection and Severity Assessment through Advanced AI Techniques

Ankita Patra, Santi Kumari Behera, Nalini Kanta Barpanda, and Prabira Kumar Sethy

8.1 INTRODUCTION

Breast cancer (BC) is a health issue that is highly prevalent worldwide and affects women. Early identification is crucial because the disease starts in cells and has the potential to spread to other parts of the body. When aberrant cells proliferate and form a mass called a lump, it is critical to identify the condition as soon as possible [1]. There are three main types of BC, all of which have different traits. The milk ducts are the exclusive site of Ductal Carcinoma In Situ (DCIS), and adjacent tissues are not invaded. Invasive Ductal Carcinoma (IDC) is the most common type in which cancer cells invade the surrounding breast tissues. The third type, Invasive Lobular Carcinoma (ILC), starts in the lobules of the milk glands and spreads to the surrounding tissues [2]. The main sign of malignant cancer is the presence of masses, which can be identified by identifying lesions that have certain characteristics related to their marginal features and structural formation. Evaluation of these masses is essential for identifying whether cancerous development is potentially malignant [3]. Notably, calcifications, deposits of calcium in the breast tissue, represent the second primary signal. In mammography images, these calcifications appear as tiny bright dots and are important diagnostic signals. To categorize cancer as benign or malignant, a thorough assessment of its physical dimensions and features is essential [4]. This entails closely examining the characteristics and structural elements of the detected masses or calcifications to determine the type of malignant development. Architectural aberrations are another important marker for BC. These distortions, which are identifiable by anomalous architectural elements, represent aberrations in the normal tissue structures. Finding these distortions is critical to the diagnosis process, as it adds to a thorough comprehension of the traits and behavior of malignancy [5]. Early diagnosis and prompt treatment are essential to lower the mortality rate of BC. Prompt intervention reduces the chance of unfavorable outcomes such as death, and early detection helps with a correct diagnosis. Customized cancer treatment, which

DOI: 10.1201/9781003469896-8

adjusts regimens for each patient, requires complex analysis at several levels, primarily related to the tumor's genetic makeup [6]. Accurate biomarker assessment is essential for making informed therapeutic decisions in breast pathology. The growing intricacy and necessity for precision in the diagnosis of histopathologic BC present difficulties, which are exacerbated by a dearth of pathologists in several regions worldwide. To improve BC diagnosis, computerized image analysis using histopathology appears to be a potential solution [7]. By expediting time-consuming processes, such as biomarker assessment, this technology may help pathologists make diagnoses that are more precise and timelier. Proactive health measures are crucial for everyone, especially women [8,9]. The likelihood of early detection and effective treatment is greatly increased by routine screening and self-examination. For patients with BC, early identification improves their quality of life by expanding their treatment options and improving their overall prognosis [10,11].

The likelihood of early detection and effective treatment is greatly increased by routine screening and self-examination. For patients with BC, early identification improves their quality of life by expanding their treatment options and improving their overall prognosis [12]. "BC can only be detected using X-rays for a considerable amount of time. A variety of imaging modalities are used to identify and assess breast abnormalities, assisting medical practitioners in making informed decisions regarding patient care". "The main objectives of BC imaging are early detection, precise diagnosis, disease staging, and therapy response monitoring. Mammography, ultrasound, magnetic resonance imaging (MRI), computed tomography (CT), positron emission tomography (PET), and three-dimensional mammography (tomosynthesis) are biomedical imaging modalities [13]". Mammography is a popular method for detecting BC. It entails obtaining X-ray images of the breast tissue to identify anomalies, such as microcalcifications or tumors. It works especially well in detecting BC in its early stages, frequently before a physical examination can detect it [14]. Sound waves are used in ultrasound to provide finely detailed images of the breast tissue. It is frequently used to separate fluid-filled cysts from solid masses or further assess abnormalities found on mammography. Breast biopsies can be more precisely targeted and sampled using ultrasound guidance [15]. Using strong magnets and radio waves, breast MRI produces detailed images of the breast. It is frequently employed in particular contexts, including high-risk individual screening, determining the severity of illness, and gauging the effectiveness of treatment. Breast MRI is especially helpful in identifying multicentric or multifocal illnesses and tiny lesions [16]. When diagnosing BC, CT scans can be helpful, particularly when assessing metastasis, the spread of the disease to other areas of the body. CT is not the primary imaging modality used to assess BC. PET scans are used in BC staging to identify distant metastases and can be used to evaluate the metabolic activity of tissues [17]. Tomosynthesis is a sophisticated type of mammography that captures pictures of the breast from various perspectives. This method reduces false positives, improves the detection of small tumors, and offers a more detailed image. Combining different imaging modalities frequently enables a more thorough evaluation of breast problems, assisting in precise diagnosis and therapeutic planning [18]. For those with BC, early detection by imaging is essential for improving prognosis and outcomes.

This paragraph explains the necessity of sophisticated AI algorithms to improve detection and severity evaluation. Large amounts of data are produced from diverse sources in industries such as healthcare, including genetic data, electronic health records, and medical photographs. These complicated data can be effectively analyzed and interpreted by advanced AI systems, assisting in the early detection of diseases and precise assessment of their severity [19]. AI systems can be trained to identify microscopic trends or abnormalities that may lead to problems. For instance, AI can help with early cancer identification in the healthcare industry, enabling prompt intervention and better results [20]. AI is vital in the age of personalized medicine. Artificial intelligence can provide customized treatment regimens by evaluating personal patient data, such as genetic information, lifestyle, and environmental factors. This increases the disease diagnosis Acc. and guarantees that each patient receives the most effective treatment, which improves outcomes [21]. Tasks that would take too much time or be impracticable for humans can now be automated owing to advanced AI capabilities. This is especially true for medical imaging, where AI can swiftly and precisely analyze hundreds of images to help radiologists diagnose ailments. Artificial intelligence (AI) in cybersecurity can automate the detection of possible threats, freeing human experts to concentrate on more difficult problems [22]. Real-time analysis is essential for many applications, including tracking the evolution of diseases and monitoring vital infrastructures. More sophisticated AI systems can continually analyze data streams, provide timely insights, and facilitate quick responses to changing conditions [23]. AI models may continuously learn from fresh data, particularly those that are ML-based. This flexibility is useful in situations in which threats or conditions change over time. For example, in cybersecurity, AI can adapt its detection algorithms based on new threat patterns [24]. In today's connected world, the amount of data collected is growing and can often be too large for conventional analytical methods. DL and other advanced AI approaches are particularly effective in handling large amounts of data because they automatically identify relevant features and patterns. This makes them ideal for jobs such as picture identification, natural language processing, and predictive analytics [25]. Because of their capacity to handle complicated data, offer early insights, personalize interventions, automate jobs, monitor in real-time, adjust to changing situations, and manage massive data effectively, advanced AI approaches are becoming increasingly necessary for detection and severity assessment [26]. These abilities support precise and effective decision-making in several crucial areas [27].

The major contributions are as follows.

- This paper consolidates findings from 125 research articles, providing a comprehensive overview of the current landscape of image-based BC detection and severity assessment.
- This review synthesizes the transformative role of AI, covering image processing, machine learning (ML), and deep learning (DL), in image-based BC detection and severity assessment.
- The paper explores the synergy between advanced image processing and ML, showcasing their combined power in automating medical image examination for nuanced BC detection.

8.2 IMAGE PROCESSING TECHNIQUES

This section comprises three sections. The different image-processing methods used for BC analysis are described in Section 8.2.1. The challenges and limitations of conventional image processing methods for BC analysis are described in Section 8.2.2. Common preprocessing techniques to enhance the quality of breast images and their comparison are presented in Section 8.2.3.

8.2.1 Image Processing Methods Used in Breast Cancer Analysis

To help diagnose BC in digital mammograms, Cahoon [28] explained the application of segmentation using fuzzy models and classification using the crisp k-nearest neighbor (k-NN) algorithm. The photos from the Digital Database for Screening Mammography (DDSM) are used in their research. We demonstrate that when intensity is the primary distinguishing characteristic, both supervised and unsupervised segmentation techniques, such as k-NN and fuzzy c-means (FCM), have significant misclassification rates in digital mammograms. The segmentations generated by the k-NN rule were (visually) improved by adding window means and standard deviations to the feature suite. Gupta et al. [29] provided an approach that involves visualizing the tumor location and determining its primary concentration. Using the Mammographic Image Analysis Society (MIAS) dataset, they extracted morphology and color information and then executed morphological procedures, such as dilatation, closing, and K Means clustering. By reducing the impact of noise, dilation using K means was used to improve the Acc. by 10%. The overall Acc. range was 60%–80%. To separate infrared breast images using heat and blood vessel activity data, Prakash et al. [30] employed three segmentation algorithms: K-Means, Fuzzy C-Means (FCM), and Gaussian Mixture Model – Expectation Maximization (GMM-EM). The strategies were then compared. FCM segmentation provides reliable diagnosis and illness indication. Younis et al. [31] used the DDMS dataset's X-ray pictures' pixels and light intensity attributes to apply a thresholding algorithm. This algorithm can be used to identify BC tumor cells. Using MIAS datasets, Varma and Sawant [32] used morphological methods like texture extraction to extract topographic features like texture and appearance. It can effectively identify BC and outline abnormalities in breast tissue. The mammography images were converted into a three-dimensional matrix. Tomar et al. [33] carry out morphological operations to extract primary radiographic signs, i.e. masses (their density, size, shape, and borders). It is effective in determining the granulometry of the tissues. Granulometry analyzes an image's object size distribution without explicitly segmenting individual objects. Using a mammography image, Sangeetha and Murthy [34] extracted brightness, contrast, size, form, and texture using a morphological operator and Otsu's thresholding technique. Ultimately, extremely early identification of the clusters allows for the classification of cancer cells as benign or malignant. Alhadidi et al. [36] compared three segmentation techniques, i.e., threshold, edge, and watershed segmentation to find BC tissue using mammography images by extracting geometric and texture features. "The threshold segmentation technique was faster than the other two segmentation methods. Adaptive histogram equalization (AHE) and morphological operations were used by Moh'd Rasoul et al. [36] to extract lymph characteristics, such as spread and intensity, from mammography X-ray images. It accurately segments each image and recognizes the area of interest in each image. To assess various parameters, such as the mean square error, peak signal-to-noise ratio, average distance, maximum difference, normalized correlation, mean absolute error, normalized error, and structural correlation, Ramani et al. [37] employed mean or average filter, median filtering, adaptive median filter, and wiener filter. Compared to other filters, the adaptive median filter [38] is a better technique for enhancing the background clarity of photos. Singh and Gupta [39] suggested a Fourier transform method to determine the stage of BC using X-ray mammography images. The frequency of dynamic infrared (IR) imaging in BC was analyzed by Joro et al. [40]". Several techniques were used. These include the Hanning window algorithm, linear image restoration techniques, high-pass filtering (HPF) with region windowing, and a Gaussian window with 2D matrix convolution. The Wiener method, which uses linear image restoration techniques, produces better results in terms of Sens. and Spec. Using the DDSM and morphological approaches such as dilatation and opening to extract texture and shape features, Helwan and Abiyev [41] achieved a 92% recognition rate for BC. Gaussian filtering was performed by Minavathi et al. [42] to extract speculation, shape, and acoustic shadows from an ultrasound image dataset. The SVM technique was then used for the classification. The algorithm's 0.88 Area Under Curve yielded 92.7% Sens. Using the MIAS breast cancer dataset, Charan et al. [43] executed morphological operations to extract image component region characteristics or regions of interest (ROI). This method aids in eliminating noise components.

Several datasets, including the DDSM [28,31,41], MIAS [29,32,43], mammographic images [32–39], dynamic infrared (IR) images [30,40], and ultrasound images [42], have been employed according to the literature survey mentioned above. Numerous approaches have been employed, including thresholding algorithms [31,35], fuzzy models [28,30], and morphological operations [29,32–34,41,43]. Table 8.1 presents various image-processing techniques for breast cancer segmentation.

8.2.2 Challenges and Limitations of Conventional Image Processing

Conventional image-processing techniques, including the detection and segmentation of breast cancer tumors, have been widely applied in the field of medical imaging. However, these techniques have several drawbacks and restrictions that have prompted researchers to investigate more complex and advanced strategies [44]. The following are some of the difficulties and restrictions that arise when traditional image processing is used for the detection and segmentation of breast cancer tumors:

- **Limited feature extraction**: When dealing with complex and heterogeneous tumors, conventional approaches may find it difficult to extract pertinent features from medical images. These techniques frequently depend on manually created features, which may not fully convey the intricacy of the pictures [45].
- **Sensitivity to image variability:** Conventional image processing methods can be affected by changes in the resolution, noise level, and contrast of the

TABLE 8.1
Different Methodologies for Breast Cancer Segmentation Using Image Processing Are Presented

References	Dataset	Image Source	Segmentation	Features	Methods	Remarks
[28]	DDSM	X-ray	Yes	Intensity by region-based features, window means	Fuzzy model, K- nearest neighbor method	K- nearest neighbor performs better
[29]	MIAS	X-ray	Yes	Morphology and color features	Morphological processes applied i.e. closing, dilation, and K means clustering	Dilation with K means has been performed to reduce the effect of noise and hence to increase the acc. by 10%. The overall acc. is 60%–80%
[30]	Infrared breast image	Photovoltaic (PV) camera	Yes	Heat, blood vessel activity	K-Means, Fuzzy C- Means (FCM) and Gaussian Mixture Model - Expectation Maximization (GMM-EM)	FCM segmentation gives good acc. and an indication of the disease
[31]	DDSM	X-ray	Yes	Pixels and light intensity	Thresholding algorithm	Breast cancer tumor detected
[32]	MIAS	X-ray	Yes	Topographic features such as texture and appearance	Morphological processes such as texture extraction	Outlining anomalies in the breast tissue and efficiently detecting breast cancer
[33]	Mammogram image and convert into 3-D matrix	X-ray	NA	Primary radiographic signs i.e. masses (their density, size, shape, borders)	Morphologic operation	Finding the granulometry of tissues
[34]	Mammographic image	X-ray	Yes	Brightness, contrast, size, shape and texture	Morphological operator and applying Otsu's thresholding algorithm	Identify the microcalcification clusters at a very early stage and classify them as benign or malignant cancer cells
[35]	Mammographic image	X-ray	Yes	Geometric and texture features	Threshold, edge, watershed segmentation	The threshold is the fastest

(Continued)

TABLE 8.1 (*Continued*)
Different Methodologies for Breast Cancer Segmentation Using Image Processing Are Presented

References	Dataset	Image Source	Segmentation	Features	Methods	Remarks
[36]	Mammographic image	X-ray	Yes	Spread, intensity, and lymph	Adaptive histogram equalization (AHE), morphological operation	Identify the region of interest and correctly segment all the images
[37]	Mammographic image	X-ray	NA	NA	Mean filter or average filter, Median filtering, adaptive median filter, wiener filter	The adaptive median filter is a more appropriate method when compared with other filters
[38]	Mammographic image converts into the 3-D matrix	X-ray	NA	NA	Fourier transform method	Detect the stage of breast cancer
[39]	Mammographic image	X-ray	Yes	Pixel intensity value	Max-mean and least-variance technique	Successful in segmenting the cancer region of mammogram
[40]	Dynamic infrared (IR) images	Photovoltaic (PV) camera	NA	NA	Gaussian window with 2D convolution of matrices, linear image restoration processes, High-pass filtering (HPF) with region windowing, Hanning window algorithm	Linear image restoration processes (the Wiener method) achieve better results
[41]	Digital database for screening mammography	X-ray	Yes	Texture and shape	Morphological techniques such as dilation and opening	The identification rate was 92%
[42]	Ultrasound image	Ultrasound	Yes	Speculation, shape, acoustic shadow	Isotropic diffusion (Gaussian filtering) and SVM	92.7% of sens. with 0.88 area under the curve
[43]	MIAS dataset	X-ray	Yes	Region of Interest (ROI), image component region	Morphological operations	Removed noise factors

acquired images. This Sens. may affect the resilience of the algorithm in various imaging modalities and environments [46].

- **Manual parameter tuning:** Many traditional techniques require manual parameter tuning, which can be laborious and difficult to modify for different datasets. Depending on the properties of the photographs, different parameter choices may be optimal [47].
- **Limited adaptability to diverse datasets:** When dealing with different datasets that vary in patient demographics, imaging modalities, and tumor types, conventional methods may not be the best fit. It is possible that they are not sufficiently adaptable to handle the underlying variability of breast cancer images [48].
- **Handling noise and artifacts:** Owing to several variables, including patient mobility and imaging equipment, medical photographs may contain noise and artifacts. Tumor segmentation Acc. may be affected if conventional approaches cannot manage and reduce these undesirable components [49].
- **Limited learning capacity:** Conventional image processing methods usually cannot automatically learn new patterns in the data. The inability to effectively generalize to previously unknown images is a potential hindrance to a robust and accurate tumor detection process [50].
- **Inability to capture spatial relationships:** The spatial relationships between pixels or voxels in an image may not be well captured by conventional approaches. This restriction may be important for applications such as tumor segmentation, where precise delineation depends on awareness of the geographical environment [51].
- **Time-consuming annotation process:** Medical picture annotation by hand is frequently labor- and expert-intensive when performed for training and validation. Annotated datasets may be a major component of conventional approaches and their production may represent a bottleneck [52].
- **Difficulty in handling large datasets:** Conventional approaches may find it difficult to interpret and analyze vast volumes of data efficiently, as medical imaging datasets continue to increase in size. This drawback may make it more difficult for them to scale and be effectively used in actual clinical settings [53].

The use of DL and ML techniques such as convolutional neural networks (CNNs) [45] and deep neural networks, which have demonstrated encouraging results in automated breast cancer tumor detection [54] and segmentation tasks [46], has changed in response to these challenges. These methods can recognize intricate patterns in medical images, adapt to a variety of datasets, and learn hierarchical characteristics directly from data.

8.2.3 Common Pre-Processing Techniques to Enhance the Quality of Breast Image

Breast photos, in particular, can be made of higher quality with the help of preprocessing techniques. These methods seek to lower noise, enhance the visibility of essential structures, and prepare photographs for precise analysis. Noise reduction

[37,62,63], contrast enhancement [55,56], image registration [64], normalization [57], image fusion [60], artifact removal [61], image cropping [58], and resizing [62], mammogram preprocessing techniques, filtering techniques, normalization, and standardization are some of the most frequently used preprocessing techniques to improve the quality of breast images.

The use of a Gaussian filter aids in lowering the high-frequency noise of the image. The median filtering technique effectively eliminates salt-and-pepper noise by substituting the value of each pixel with the median value of its surrounding area. By redistributing the image intensity levels, the histogram equalization approach improves the overall contrast. By enhancing the local contrast, contrast-limited adaptive histogram equalization (CLAHE) prevents noise in homogeneous regions from being too amplified. Several photos taken at various periods or with various modalities may be registered to enhance the overall quality and facilitate comparison analysis. Maintaining constant intensity levels between various modalities or images contributes to the increased comparability of the images. Integrating data from various imaging modalities (such as mammography and MRI) can yield a more thorough picture of breast tissue. Accurate diagnosis depends on the correction of imaging artifacts such as motion artifacts and equipment-related artifacts. The effectiveness of the analysis can be increased by concentrating on the pertinent breast region and eliminating extraneous backdrops. Changing the image resolution can aid in standardizing data for subsequent processing. The pectoral muscle region can be removed to enhance breast tissue visibility in mammograms. Early detection can be facilitated by emphasizing microcalcifications, which are suggestive of specific disorders. Improving the image's edges can help make the boundaries between various components easier to see. Additionally, a new field of study in medical imaging is the application of deep-learning-based techniques for picture augmentation. A state-of-the-art comparison of several preprocessing techniques and their outcomes are presented in Table 8.2.

8.3 APPLICATION OF MACHINE LEARNING FOR BREAST CANCER DETECTION

ML has demonstrated considerable potential in the identification and diagnosis of breast cancer. Large databases of clinical data and medical imaging can be analyzed using ML algorithms to facilitate early diagnosis, risk assessment, and therapy planning. By helping radiologists identify worrisome spots in mammograms, ML algorithms can increase the precision of breast cancer screening. DL architectures, such as CNNs, can be trained to recognize irregularities and subtle patterns in mammograms. Between various preprocessing techniques and their outcomes, ML algorithms can segment and identify lesions in breast MRI and ultrasound images, offering more precise information for diagnosis. To help characterize the type of observed anomalies, ML models can be used to analyze the textural properties of lesions. By examining a variety of variables, including genetic information, family history, and clinical data, ML algorithms can determine an individual's risk of developing breast cancer. By customizing treatment regimens based on each patient's unique features, ML can maximize the efficacy of therapies.

TABLE 8.2
Different Breast Cancer Image Preprocessing Methodologies and their Results

Reference	Motive	Proposed Model	Parameter Evaluation	Remarks
[37]	To remove special markings and unwanted noises	Mean filter or average filter, median filtering, adaptive median filter, wiener filter	Mean square error, peak signal – to – noise-ratio, structural content	The adaptive median filter is better when compared with the other filter
[55]	To improve the detection quality of breast cancer	Median, wiener, and anisotropic filtering with wavelet	Acc. is examined in terms of standard deviation (SD), peak signal-to-noise ratio (PSNR), signal-to-noise ratio (SNR), self-similarity index measure (SSIM), IMAE, VAR, Root Mean Square Error (RMSE), AMBE	Anisotropic filtering with wavelet can produce significantly improved results (qualitatively and quantitatively) as compared to other filtering methods
[56]	To improve image quality for analysis (breast periphery separation, intensity ratio propagation, breast thickness estimation, and intensity balancing	Otsu binary segmentation, Morphological operation	Acc.	Useful in quantifying change in the relative proportion of breast tissue
[57]	To remove the background area (high-intensity rectangular label, tape artifact, and noise)	Contrast stretching, Two dimensional (2D) Median Filtering	Peak Signal to Noise Ratio (PSNR)	Thresholds and regions of segmentation algorithms work more efficiently when images are pre-processed
[58]	Background removal, and image enhancements to outline the ROIs and regions within the ROIs	Rolling Ball Algorithm, Huang's Fuzzy Thresholding, Canny Edge Detection, and Hough's Line Transform	Acc., mean gray value and the standard deviation, mean squared error, peak signal-to-noise-ratio, structural similarity index measure	Artifacts and noise are removed from the images

(*Continued*)

TABLE 8.2 (*Continued*)
Different Breast Cancer Image Preprocessing Methodologies and their Results

Reference	Motive	Proposed Model	Parameter Evaluation	Remarks
[59]	A technique producing higher detectability of lesions	Filtered-back projection (FBP) algorithm	Detectability index	Breast border enhancement artifacts were greatly suppressed and the detectability of calcifications and masses was increased
[60]	Develop an automated system for assisting in the analysis of digital mammograms	Edge-based segmentation, Poisson-based region segmentation	Evaluate each pixel in the image and compare it to the other pixels to determine distinct groups	Accurately detect the region of interest (ROI) for pectoral muscle, suppress the pectoral muscle successfully
[61]	Identification of suspicious lesions and micro-calcifications	Contrast Stretching, power-law transformation, histogram processing, un-sharp masking, morphological processing, median filtering, anisotropic diffusion filtering, bilateral enhancement, homomorphic filtering	Peak Signal to Noise Ratio (PSNR)	Anisotropic diffusion, power-law transformation, un-sharp masking, morphological processing, and median filtering are giving higher PSNR values
[62]	To detect the region of interest, automatic removal of artifacts and noise	Otsu's N thresholding method, threshold-based segmentation, edge-based segmentation, region-based segmentation	Mean Square Error (MSE), Peak Signal-to-Noise Ratio (PSNR), enhancement measure (EME)	Otsu's N thresholding is better than another thresholding method
[63]	Enhance image quality, image smoothing, and noise restoration	Adaptive weighted frost filter for quantum noise removal	Spatial resolution, Peak Signal to Noise Ratio (PSNR)	Adaptive Weighted Frost filter is the most suitable choice for eliminating noise from mammographic images and performs better comparatively
[64]	Highlighting the required features of the image and suppressing noises	CNN architecture	Acc.	Cleaning of the noises and drying of the properties

Using the Wisconsin Diagnosis Breast Cancer (WDBC) dataset, Sharma et al. [65] presented several ML algorithms, including RF, K-nearest neighbor, and naïve Bayes, to categorize benign and malignant breast cancer tumors. After assessing recall, Acc., precision, and f1 score, it was discovered that KNN performed the best for classification. "Using the same dataset to classify two different types of breast cancer, Benign and Malignant, Bazazeh and Shubair [66] used support vector machines (SVM), RFs, and Bayesian networks. They also evaluated the Acc., recall, precision, and area of the response curve (ROC)". The RF technique offers the best ROC performance, whereas the Bayesian Network (BN) performs best in terms of recall and precision. "Using ML techniques, such as RF, KNN, Naïve Bayes, SVM, and RF, Ak [67] created a model to identify breast cancer and determine accuracy. The LR model that contained all features produced the best results, with a classification Acc. of 98.1%." In their study, Vaka et al. [68] examined and contrasted threshold, DNSS, FCM, and histo-sigmoid fuzzy clustering. The DNNS was determined to be far superior to current techniques. To identify breast cancer with high accuracy, Alarabeyyat and Alhanahnah [69] created a Backpropagation Neural Network (BPNN), LR, and the Backpropagation neural Network using mammography pictures to evaluate the number of features that are extracted. Compared with the BPNN, the LR model used a significantly larger number of characteristics. SVM-RBF provided the highest overall Acc. of 96.33%. Nallamala et al. [71] suggested the LR Algorithm, SVM Algorithm, and KNN Algorithm classify two different kinds of breast cancer tumors, i.e., Benign and Malignant using mammography images. Osareh and Shadgar [70] used SVM, KNN, and PNN models to distinguish between the benign and malignant tumors of the breast using fine needle aspirates of breast lesions and fine needle aspirates of breast lumps (FNAB). They also compared performance metrics such as Acc., Sens., Spec., and MCC. The proposed method assesses yield decipherability, computation time, and predictive capability. The proposed model achieved 98.1% Acc. Using the University of California, Irvine (UCI) ML library, Omondiagbe et al. [72] used RBF, ANN, and Naïve Bayes classifiers in conjunction with SVM to extract features and minimize their dimensions. SVM achieved a maximum classification Acc. of 98.82%, Sens. of 98.41%, Spec. of 99.07%, and area under the receiver operating characteristic curve of 0.9994, according to calculations of Acc., the area under the ROC curve, precision, recall, Sens., Spec., and kappa statistic. The proposed method assesses yield decipherability, computation time, and predictive capability. The proposed model achieved 98.1% accuracy. Using the University of California, Irvine (UCI) ML library, Omondiagbe et al. [72] used RBF, ANN, and Naïve Bayes classifiers in conjunction with SVM to extract features and minimize their dimensions. SVM achieved a maximum classification Acc. of 98.82%, Sens. of 98.41%, Spec. of 99.07%, and area under the receiver operating characteristic curve of 0.9994, according to calculations of Acc., the area under the ROC curve, precision, recall, Sens., Spec., and kappa statistic. The MLP model performed the best in terms of Acc., precision, and recall of 99.12%, 99.00%, and 99.00%, respectively, after comparing the Acc., precision, and recall of the classification tests. "To automatically detect breast cancer using an ML algorithm using the Wisconsin Breast Cancer dataset, Dhahri et al. [76] adopted SVM, KNN, DT, gradient boosting classifier (GB), RF, LR, AdaBoost classifier (AB), Gaussian Naive Bayes (GNB), and LDA models." After comparing performance metrics such as Acc., recall, precision, and f1 score, it can be determined that, with appropriate configuration, the algorithms will perform identically. Using the WDBC dataset, Safdar et al. [77] compared ML algorithms to accurately predict breast cancer detection. After evaluating the AUC and receiver operating curve (ROC), it was discovered that KNN outperformed SVM. "Radial Based Function, Simple Linear LR Model, Naïve Bayes, k-Nearest Neighbour, AdaBoost, Fuzzy Unordered Role Induction technique, DT - J48, SVM, and WBCD datasets were employed by Gbenga et al. [78] in the identification of breast cancer." After calculating the TPR, FPR, precision, F1 score, and Acc., it was discovered that the SVM outperformed the others. Using the DDMS dataset, Hussain et al. compared Bayesian, SVM, and decision-tree classifier models. The Acc., Sens., Spec., and FPR were computed. SVM had the lowest FPR, maximum Sens., Spec., and Acc. A state-of-the-art comparison of various ML models for the diagnosis and categorization of breast cancer illnesses is presented in Table 8.3.

8.4 EMERGENCE OF DEEP LEARNING IN BREAST CANCER IMAGING

In the field of breast cancer imaging, DL has advanced significantly and offers promising improvements in diagnosis, treatment, and detection. The analysis of mammograms using DL models has aided the early detection of breast cancer. These models are capable of identifying minute patterns and anomalies that human radiologists can find difficult to recognize. By autonomously identifying and segmenting breast lesions in medical photographs, DL algorithms can expedite diagnosis and lower the risk of human error. Histopathological images of breast tissue can be analyzed using DL algorithms to categorize various subtypes of breast cancer. Appropriate treatment plans must be determined using this information. In the field of breast cancer imaging, DL has advanced significantly and offers promising improvements in diagnosis, treatment, and detection. The analysis of mammograms using DL models has aided the early detection of breast cancer. These models are capable of identifying minute patterns and anomalies that human radiologists can find difficult to recognize. By autonomously identifying and segmenting breast lesions in medical photographs, DL algorithms can expedite diagnosis and lower the risk of human error. Histopathological images of breast tissue can be analyzed using DL algorithms to categorize various subtypes of breast cancer. Appropriate treatment plans must be determined using this information. By lowering the false positives and negatives in breast cancer imaging, DL models seek to increase the overall diagnosis Acc. This is especially crucial for reducing pointless interventions and ensuring that patients receive timely therapy. The speed and Acc. of breast cancer screening programs can be increased by integrating DL algorithms into CAD systems to help radiologists interpret screening mammograms. DL in breast cancer imaging has the potential to significantly enhance personalized treatment plans, early diagnosis, and early detection, all of which can improve patient outcomes. To address these issues and guarantee the responsible application of new technologies in healthcare, continued research and cooperation among physicians, data scientists, and regulatory agencies is important.

TABLE 8.3
Comparison of Machine Learning Models for Breast Cancer Disease Identification and Classification

Reference	Dataset	Motive	Algorithms/Techniques Used	Parameter Evaluation	Results
[65]	Wisconsin Diagnosis Breast Cancer (WDBC)	To train and test models to classify two different kinds of breast cancer i.e., Benign and Malignant	RF, KNN and Naïve Bayes	Acc., precision, recall, and F1 score	k-NN is the most effective in the detection of breast cancer with 94% accuracy
[66]	Wisconsin Diagnosis Breast Cancer (WDBC)	To classify two different kinds of breast cancer i.e., Benign and Malignant	SVM, RF and Bayesian Networks (BN)	Acc., recall, precision, and area of ROC	Bayesian Network (BN) has the best performance in terms of recall and precision, RF technique has the optimum ROC performance
[67]	Wisconsin Diagnosis Breast Cancer (WDBC)	To detect breast cancer	RF, KNN, Naïve Bayes, and SVM	Acc.	Results obtained with the LR model with all features included showed the highest classification Acc. (98.1%)
[68]	M. G Cancer Hospital & Research Institute, Visakhapatnam	To detect breast cancer	Histo-sigmoid fuzzy clustering, DNSS, FCM, threshold	Acc.	DNNS is quite better than the existing methods
[69]	Mammography image	To detect breast cancer with high acc.	Backpropagation Neural Network (BPNN), LR, and the Backpropagation Neural Network	Numbers of features	The number of features utilized in the LR model was much higher than with the BPNN
[70]	Fine needle aspirate of breast lesions, fine needle aspirates of breast lumps (FNAB)	To distinguish between the benign and malignant tumors of the breast	SVM, KNN, PNN	Acc., sens., spec., MCC	SVM-RBF provided the highest overall Acc. of 96.33%
[71]	Mammography Image	To classify two different kinds of breast cancer tumors i.e., Benign and Malignant	LR Algorithm, SVM Algorithm, KNN Algorithm	Ease to decipher yield, calculation time, and predictive power	The suggested strategy has acquired 98.50% precision

(Continued)

TABLE 8.3 (*Continued*)
Comparison of Machine Learning Models for Breast Cancer Disease Identification and Classification

Reference	Dataset	Motive	Algorithms/Techniques Used	Parameter Evaluation	Results
[72]	University of California-Irvine (UCI) ML repository	Feature selection and feature extraction methods to reduce the dimension of features	SVM with RBF, ANN, and Naïve Bayes classifier	Acc., area under ROC curve, precision, recall, sens., spec., kappa statistic	SVM achieves classification acc. of 98.82%, Sens. of 98.41%, spec. of 99.07%, and area under the receiver operating characteristic curve of 0.9994
[73]	Mammography image	To detect breast cancer tumor	SVM, ANN, KNN, DT	Acc., sens., spec., MCC	The maximum achieved acc. of SVM (single or hybrid) was 99.8%
[74]	BreakHist_Dataset	To distinguish between malignant and benign tumor	SVM, RF, KNN, LR, Naïve Bayes	Identify specific parts using specific filters	KNN outperforms other methods
[75]	Wisconsin Diagnosis Breast Cancer (WDBC)	Evaluate the performance in classifying data concerning the efficiency and effectiveness of each algorithm	MLP, KNN, Classification and Regression Trees (CART), Gaussian Nave Bayes (NB) and SVMs	Classification tests acc., precision, and recall	MLP model has the highest performance in terms of acc., precision, and recall at 99.12%, 99.00%, and 99.00% respectively
[76]	Wisconsin Breast Cancer dataset	Automatic detection of breast cancer using an ML algorithm	SVM, KNN, DT, gradient boosting classifier (GB), RF, LR, AdaBoost classifier (AB), Gaussian Naive Bayes (GNB), and LDA	Acc., recall, prec., F1 score	The algorithms can achieve the same performance after effective configuration
[77]	Breast Cancer Wisconsin Diagnostic Dataset (BCWD)	Comparing ML models for correctly predicting breast cancer detection	SVM, LR, and KNN	Receiver-operating curve (ROC), and the AUC evaluate a classifier for precise acc.	Overall average Acc. of KNN is higher than SVM
[78]	Wisconsin breast cancer datasets	Detection of breast cancer	Radial Based Function, Simple Linear LR Model, Naïve Bayes, KNN, AdaBoost, Fuzzy Unordered Role Induction algorithm and DT - J48, SVM	TPR, FPR, Precision, F1 score, acc.	SVM has the best performance in terms of classification acc. and the lowest FR
[79]	Digital Database for Screening Mammography (DDMS)	To distinguish the cancer mammograms	SVM, DT, and Bayesian classifier	Acc., sens., spec., FPR	SVM has the highest acc., sens., spec., and lowest FPR

To assess the AUC, Sens., and Spec., Shen et al. [79] suggested utilizing VGG16 and ResNet 50-based image classification to classify breast cancer using mammogram images using the DDSM (CBIS-DDSM). ResNet50 performed the best. The relative values of the AUC, Sens., and Spec. were 98%, 86.7%, and 96.1%, respectively. Utilizing strong computer vision techniques and DL models, Mambou et al. [81] evaluated linear SVM and InceptionV3 for numerous breast cancer diagnosis strategies utilizing a research database (DMR) comprising frontal thermogram images and calculated Acc. and AUC. In comparison, SVM performs better than the others. "Using the IRMA dataset, Ismail and Sovuthy [81] created VGG16 and ResNet50 to test the diagnosis of breast cancer between two DL model networks. The optimal model, VGG16, had an Acc. of 94%, precision of 89%, and recall of 99%. The efficient Adaboost algorithm (DLA-EABA) for breast cancer detection utilizing MRI images was proposed by Zheng et al. [82]. It attains 97.2% Acc., 98.3% Sens., and 96.5% Spec.." Using synthetic datasets and image datasets related to breast histopathology, Das et al. [83] presented 2-DEWT decomposed modes by transforming a one-dimensional signal into two-dimensional images using the deep insight framework and the mean normalization technique. Using full-field digital mammography (FFDM), Bai et al. [84] built and compared deep and recurrent neural networks to identify malignancies before clinical indications manifest. It was found that the Acc., Sens., Spec., and precision of the deep neural networks were all higher. Optimized feature extraction and selection were carried out by Sha et al. [85] using the grasshopper optimization method. Before processing, a median filter was used to remove noise from the image and optimize image segmentation using the CNN and DDSM databases. It attained 92% Acc., 97% NPV, 85% PPV, 93% Spec., and 96% Sens. Lotter et al. [86] Using an annotation-efficient DL approach with DDSM pictures, new "maximum suspicion projection" (MSP) images were created from DBT data to detect mammography and digital breast tomosynthesis. It attained a Sens. of 97.7%, Spec. of 99.4% and AUC of 0.963 ± 0.003. Using the mammography MIAS database, Khuriwal and Mishra [87] created a CNN to detect breast cancer from histological pictures. The CNN approach achieved 98% Acc. for the 12 features. CNNs were proposed by Salvi and Kadam [89] for the identification of breast cancer using thermal camera sensor image datasets. Using this method, a 98% Acc. was attained. O-net, a mixture of two U-nets connected at the encoding level and disconnected at the decoding level, was developed by Rashed and El Seoud [89] to develop an automated breast cancer diagnosis system employing mammography and the CBIS-DDSM dataset. The Acc. is 95.01%. In a study conducted by Selvathi and Poornila [90], breast cancer diagnosis utilizing medical images and the MIAS mammography dataset was compared using CNNs, sparse autoencoders (SAE), and supervised SAEs (SSAE). GoogleNet, AlexNet, VGG16, and FaceNet were examined by Wang et al. [91] to identify metastatic breast cancer from histopathological images. The Acc. rates for GoogleNet, AlexNet, VGG16, and faceNet are 98.4%, 92.1%, 97.9%, and 96.8%, respectively. With a 99.67% Acc. rate, Khuriwal and Mishra [92] suggested a CNN for breast cancer diagnosis utilizing a DL algorithm and the Wisconsin Breast Cancer Database. Using the CBIS-DDSM dataset, Ragab et al. [93] employed SVMs and deep CNNs for the diagnosis of breast cancer. SVM obtained an AUC of 94% and an Acc. of 87.2%. Khan et al. [94] used the idea of transfer learning with a standard benchmark dataset to compare GoogleNet, VGGNet, and ResNet for the detection and classification of breast cancer. The accuracies of GoogleNet, VGGNet, and ResNet are 93.5%, 94.15%, and 94.35%, respectively. Using the MIAS dataset. Saber et al. [95] compared Inception V3, ResNet50, VGG-16, VGG-19, and Inception-V2 ResNet. More power is present in the VGG16 model. The F1-score, AUC, Sens., Spec., Acc., and precision were 98.56%, 97.25%, 97.66%, 99.5%, and 98.96%, respectively. A comparison of the various DL models for breast cancer diagnosis is presented in Table 8.4.

8.5 INTEGRATION OF IMAGING AND AI IN BREAST CANCER DIAGNOSIS

The combination of artificial intelligence (AI) [96] with imaging for the diagnosis of breast cancer has demonstrated great potential in terms of enhancing the precision, effectiveness, and customized nature of diagnostic procedures.

- **Automated image analysis:** Mammograms and tomosynthesis photos were analyzed using AI algorithms to identify anomalies such as masses, microcalcifications, and architectural distortions [97]. Radiologists can benefit from automated analysis because it shortens interpretation times and highlights areas of concern.
- **MRI and ultrasound analysis:** Artificial intelligence was utilized to evaluate breast MRI and ultrasound images, offering further data for diagnosis. This covers the distinction between benign and malignant signs, as well as the identification of lesions and characterization of tumors [98].
- **Computer-Aided Detection (CAD):** AI-driven computer-aided design (CAD) systems have been created to assist radiologists in interpreting images. By marking possible regions of interest, these technologies help radiologists identify anomalies that can be difficult to notice or easily missed [99].
- **Quantitative imaging biomarkers:** Through radiomics analysis, AI makes it easier to extract quantitative characteristics from medical images. These traits function as imaging biomarkers and offer important insights into the properties and behavior of tumors [100]. Imaging for breast cancer can be made more diagnostic and prognostic by using radiomics.
- **Integration with clinical data:** Imaging data can be integrated with clinical, genetic, and other patient-specific data using artificial intelligence [51]. This all-encompassing method improves diagnostic precision and aids in customized treatment planning.
- **Risk stratification:** To categorize patients into distinct risk groups, AI models can evaluate a variety of risk variables and imaging findings [101]. This will facilitate the creation of customized management plans and suitable screening intervals.
- **Real-time decision support:** A CDSS driven by AI [102] helps radiologists assess images in real time. It can provide advice based on imaging data analysis, and assist medical professionals in making better judgments.

TABLE 8.4
Comparison of Different Deep-Learning Models for Breast Cancer Detection

Reference	Dataset	Motive	Algorithms / Techniques Used	Parameter Evaluation	Results
[80]	DDSM	To classify breast cancer using mammogram images	VGG16 and ResNet50-based image classification	AUC, sens., spec.	ResNet50 shows the best performance. AUC: 0.98, sens.: 86.7% and spec.: 96.1%
[81]	Research Data Base (DMR) containing frontal thermogram images	Comparative study of several breast cancer detection techniques using powerful computer vision techniques and DL models	Linear SVM, InceptionV3	Acc., AUC	SVM is comparatively better than others
[82]	IRMA dataset	Compare breast cancer detection with two model networks of DL techniques	VGG16 and ResNet50	Acc., precision. recall	VGG16 performs best. acc.: 94%, precision: 89%, recall: 99%
[83]	MRI image	Breast cancer detection	Efficient Adaboost Algorithm (DLA-EABA)	Acc., sens., spec.	Acc.: 97.2%, sens.: 98.3%, spec.: 96.5%
[84]	Synthetic datasets and breast histopathology image datasets	Converting the one-dimensional signal to two-dimensional images using the deep insight framework with the mean normalization technique	2-DEWT decomposed modes	Acc., Sens., Spec., Precision, Recall, F1score	Acc.: 98.08%, sens.: 99.20%, spec.: 93.55%, precision: 98.41%, recall: 99.20%, F1score: 98.80%

(*Continued*)

TABLE 8.4 (*Continued*)
Comparison of Different Deep-Learning Models for Breast Cancer Detection

Reference	Dataset	Motive	Algorithms / Techniques Used	Parameter Evaluation	Results
[85]	Full-field digital mammography (FFDM)	Identification of cancers before clinical signs appear	Deep Neural Networks, Autoencoders, Deep CNN, RNN and Generative Adversarial Networks	Acc., false positive rate, precision, recall, F1 score, ROC curve, AUC, Precision-Recall	FFDMs, deep-learning–based detection is the most effective models
[86]	DDSM	Pre-processed by a median filter for noise elimination, and optimized image segmentation based on a CNN	A grasshopper optimization algorithm, and optimized feature extraction and feature selection based on the grasshopper optimization algorithm	Acc., sens., spec., NPV, PPV	96% sens., 93% spec., 85% PPV, 97% NPV, 92% acc.
[87]	DDSM	Detection in mammography and digital breast tomosynthesis using an annotation-efficient DL approach	Creating new 'maximum suspicion projection' (MSP) images from DBT data	AUC, sens., spec.	AUC: 0.963 ± 0.003, sens.: 97.7%, spec.: 99.4%
[88]	Mammograph MIAS database	Breast cancer detection from histopathological images	CNN	Acc.	CNN algorithm on these 12 features and achieved 98% acc.
[89]	Thermal camera sensor	Breast cancer detection	CNN	Acc.	Acc.: 98%
[90]	Curated Breast Imaging Subset (CBIS-DDSM)	Development of an automatic diagnosis system for breast cancer using mammography	O-net, which is a combination of two U-nets connected at the encoding level and disconnected at the decoding	Acc.	Acc.: 95.01%
[91]	Mini-MIAS mammographic database	Breast cancer detection using medical image	CNN, sparse autoencoder (SAE), supervised SAE(SSAE)	Acc.	Acc. of up to 97%, 98.5% for SAE, 98.9% for SSAE

(Continued)

TABLE 8.4 (*Continued*)
Comparison of Different Deep-Learning Models for Breast Cancer Detection

Reference	Dataset	Motive	Algorithms / Techniques Used	Parameter Evaluation	Results
[92]	Histopathology image	Identifying metastatic breast cancer	GoogleNet, AlexNet, VGG16, FaceNet	Acc.	GoogleNet: 98.4%, AlexNet: 92.1%, VGG16: 97.9%, FaceNet: 96.8%
[93]	Wisconsin breast cancer database	Breast cancer diagnosis using DL algorithm	CNN	Acc.	Acc.: 99.67%.
[94]	Curated Breast Imaging Subset of DDSM (CBIS-DDSM)	Breast cancer detection	Deep CNN and SVMs	Acc., AUC	SVM acc. becomes 87.2% with an AUC equaling 0.94 (94%)
[95]	Standard benchmark dataset	Detection and classification of breast cancer using the concept of transfer learning	GoogleNet, VGGNet, and ResNet	Acc.	Acc. of GoogleNet, VGGNet, and ResNet are 93.5%, 94.15%, and 94.35% respectively
[96]	MIAS dataset	Acc., sens., spec., precision, F-score, and AUC	Inception V3, ResNet50, Visual Geometry Group networks (VGG)-19, VGG-16, and Inception-V2 ResNet.	Acc., sens., spec., precision, F-score, and AUC	VGG16 model is powerful. Acc., Sens., Spec., precision, F-score, and AUC are 98.96%, 97.83%, 99.13%, 97.35%, 97.66%, and 0.995, respectively

- **Telemedicine and remote consultation:** AI makes it easier to transmit and analyze imaging data remotely, allowing specialists and healthcare professionals to collaborate. This is especially helpful in places where access to qualified radiologists is scarce [103].
- **Continuous learning and model improvement:** AI models constantly learn and change in response to fresh information and new trends [104]. Over time, this flexibility helps algorithms perform better and keeps them up-to-date with the most recent advancements in imaging methods and medical understanding.

8.6 IMPACT ON CLINICAL DECISION MAKING

Clinical decision-making in breast cancer has been significantly affected by the combination of AI and image processing. AI algorithms can improve the Sens. and Spec. of breast cancer detection in medical images such as mammograms and MRIs [105]. This advancement facilitates early diagnosis and improves treatment outcomes. By automatically indicating any anomalies or suspicious areas in medical images, AI-based CAD [106] systems help radiologists. This can improve the diagnosis Acc. and decrease oversight. AI makes it possible to extract and analyze quantitative features from medical images through radiomics. These traits function as imaging biomarkers [107] and offer more details regarding the nature of tumors. A more accurate diagnosis and prognosis can be achieved using radiomics. To estimate a patient's chance of acquiring breast cancer, AI models can examine a variety of imaging data, medical history, and other pertinent data [108]. Customizing screening methods and choosing appropriate therapies are made easier with the use of this information. AI systems can assist in the creation of individualized treatment regimens by predicting molecular subtypes of breast cancer based on imaging characteristics. This method assists medical professionals in selecting treatments with a higher chance of working for particular subtypes. AI can be used to track how a tumor's properties and response to treatment vary over time. These data will help medical professionals modify their treatment plans according to each patient's reaction to therapy. AI makes it easier to combine genomic and clinical data with the imaging data. Clinical decision support systems (CDSS) driven by AI [109] can help physicians make decisions in real time by recommending and supplying pertinent data. This helps medical practitioners make judgments faster and with greater Acc. By automating repetitive and time-consuming operations, AI allows healthcare personnel to concentrate on more intricate patient care responsibilities. Faster diagnosis and treatment initiation may result in increased efficiency [110]. AI makes it easier for specialists to analyze medical images remotely, allowing them to counsel and assist medical practitioners who are located in different locations [111]. This is particularly helpful in places where access to specialized knowledge is scarce. The use of AI and image processing technologies in breast cancer clinical decision-making has many advantages; however, to ensure their safe and successful integration into standard clinical practice, it is critical to address issues such as data privacy, the interpretability of AI models, and ongoing validation [112]. Encouraging research, cooperation, and regulatory supervision is necessary to fully utilize these technologies for the treatment of breast cancer.

8.7 CHALLENGES AND FUTURE DIRECTIONS

Caliber and variety of training data have a significant impact on the effectiveness of AI models. Problems such as unbalanced datasets and differences in imaging methods can affect the generalizability of the models. Clinicians frequently need transparent insights into the decision-making process; hence, the absence of interpretability and explainability in AI models is a barrier [113]. It is difficult to seamlessly integrate AI technologies into current clinical operations. The adoption of AI technologies may be hampered by interoperability problems, resistance to change, and concerns regarding disruption. The effectiveness of AI algorithms may be affected by variations in image quality and format caused by the absence of uniform imaging practices throughout healthcare facilities [114]. Complicated issues surround informed permission, patient privacy, and the ethical application of AI in healthcare. Legal and ethical frameworks must be developed in parallel with new technological development.

AI models can be made more robust and reliable by incorporating real-world clinical data and carefully selecting various relevant datasets [115]. Ongoing studies to create models and explanation methods for AI forecasts that are easier to understand. Gaining trust and easing the incorporation of AI into clinical workflows are needed [116]. To provide user-friendly interfaces, guarantee interoperability with current systems, and provide comprehensive training for healthcare personnel, technologists, and healthcare professionals to collaborate [117]. The promotion and creation of standardized imaging procedures to guarantee uniformity in data collection may improve the ability of AI models to generalize in various contexts. Defining precise privacy protection, ethical standards [118], and legal frameworks to control the advancement and application of AI in breast cancer diagnosis. It is imperative to guarantee patient participation in the decision-making procedures [119].

8.8 CONCLUSION

A revolutionary era in the identification and assessment of breast cancer severity has been brought about by the combination of sophisticated AI tools and image-based methods. The transition from conventional techniques to AI-powered technologies have shown revolutionary changes in breast cancer diagnosis. These technologies have demonstrated greater skill in identifying minor abnormalities, supporting early detection, and offering insights into the severity of breast cancer through the application of ML and DL algorithms. AI integration helps radiologists plan treatments more precisely and individually while also increasing their productivity. Obstacles such as data integrity, comprehensibility, and moral implications highlight the necessity of continuous investigation and cooperation. The field will advance further with the support of explainable AI, multimodal integration, and international data-sharing initiatives, promising more accurate, effective, and patient-centered care for breast cancer patients. The combination of AI with image-based approaches has yielded transformative discoveries that represent a paradigm shift in breast cancer management. These insights have the potential to significantly improve outcomes and eventually save lives.

FUNDING

This research is not funded by any organization.

CONFLICT OF INTEREST

The authors have no conflict of interest.

REFERENCES

1. Ye, Feng, et al. "Advancements in clinical aspects of targeted therapy and immunotherapy in breast cancer." *Molecular Cancer* 22.1 (2023): 105.
2. Rakha, Emad A., Gary M. Tse, and Cecily M. Quinn. "An update on the pathological classification of breast cancer." *Histopathology* 82.1 (2023): 5–16.
3. Subhan, Md Abdus, et al. "Recent advances with precision medicine treatment for breast cancer including triple-negative sub-type." *Cancers* 15.8 (2023): 2204.
4. Guo, Liantao, et al. "Breast cancer heterogeneity and its implication in personalized precision therapy." *Experimental Hematology & Oncology* 12.1 (2023): 1–27.
5. Nolan, Emma, Geoffrey J. Lindeman, and Jane E. Visvader. "Deciphering breast cancer: From biology to the clinic." *Cell* 186.8 (2023): 1708–1728.
6. Tariq, Mehreen, et al. "Medical image-based breast cancer diagnosis: State of the art and future directions." *Expert Systems with Applications* 167 (2021): 114095.
7. Zhang, Ya-nan, et al. "Review of breast cancer pathological image processing." *BioMed Research International* 2021 (2021): 1–7.
8. Robertson, Stephanie, et al. "Digital image analysis in breast pathology—From image processing techniques to Artificial Intelligence." *Translational Research* 194 (2018): 19–35.
9. Yasmin, Mussarat, Muhammad Sharif, and Sajjad Mohsin. "Survey paper on diagnosis of breast cancer using image processing techniques." *Reseach Journal of Recent Sciences* 2.10(2013): 88–98. ISSN 2277-2502.
10. Veta, Mitko, et al. "Breast cancer histopathology image analysis: A review." *IEEE Transactions on Biomedical Engineering* 61.5 (2014): 1400–1411.
11. Gayathri, B. K., and P. Raajan. "A survey of breast cancer detection based on image segmentation techniques." *2016 International Conference on Computing Technologies and Intelligent Data Engineering (ICCTIDE'16)*. IEEE, Kovilpatti, India, 2016.
12. Lin, Hairong, et al. "Brain-like initial-boosted hyperchaos and application in biomedical image encryption." *IEEE Transactions on Industrial Informatics* 18.12 (2022): 8839–8850.
13. Chen, Ying, Shangfeng Wang, and Fan Zhang. "Near-infrared luminescence high-contrast in vivo biomedical imaging." *Nature Reviews Bioengineering* 1.1 (2023): 60–78.
14. Rivera-Fernández, Josué D., et al. "Design of a low-cost diffuse optical mammography system for biomedical image processing in breast cancer diagnosis." *Sensors* 23.9 (2023): 4390.
15. Li, Jiapu, et al. "Recent advancements in ultrasound transducer: From material strategies to biomedical applications." *BME Frontiers* 2022 (2022): 9764501.
16. Al Ewaidat, Haytham, and Mohammad Ayasrah. "A concise review on the utilization of abbreviated protocol breast MRI over full diagnostic protocol in breast cancer detection." *International Journal of Biomedical Imaging* 2022 (2022): 8705531.
17. Nazari, Mahsa, et al. "Current status and future prospects of nanoscale metal–organic frameworks in bioimaging." *Journal of Materials Chemistry B* 10.43 (2022): 8824–8851.

18. Iqbal, Ahmed, et al. "Generative adversarial networks and its applications in the biomedical image segmentation: A comprehensive survey." *International Journal of Multimedia Information Retrieval* 11.3 (2022): 333–368.
19. Acosta, Julián N., et al. "Multimodal biomedical AI." *Nature Medicine* 28.9 (2022): 1773–1784.
20. Gichoya, Judy Wawira, et al. "AI recognition of patient race in medical imaging: A modeling study." *The Lancet Digital Health* 4.6 (2022): e406–e414.
21. Tu, Tao, et al. "Towards generalist biomedical AI." *arXiv preprint arXiv:2307.14334* (2023).
22. Chen, Haomin, et al. "Explainable medical imaging AI needs human-centered design: Guidelines and evidence from a systematic review." *NPJ Digital Medicine* 5.1 (2022): 156.
23. Soomro, Toufique A., et al. "Artificial Intelligence (AI) for medical imaging to combat coronavirus disease (COVID-19): A detailed review with direction for future research." *Artificial Intelligence Review* 55 (2022): 1409–1439.
24. Yousefirizi, Fereshteh, et al. "AI-based detection, classification and prediction/prognosis in medical imaging: Towards radiophenomics." *PET Clinics* 17.1 (2022): 183–212.
25. Holzinger, Andreas, et al. "AI for life: Trends in Artificial Intelligence for biotechnology." *New Biotechnology* 74 (2023): 16–24.
26. Kaviani, Sara, Ki Jin Han, and Insoo Sohn. "Adversarial attacks and defenses on AI in medical imaging informatics: A survey." *Expert Systems with Applications* 198 (2022): 116815.
27. King, Michael R. "The future of AI in medicine: A perspective from a Chatbot." *Annals of Biomedical Engineering* 51.2 (2023): 291–295.
28. Cahoon, Tobias Christian, Melanie A. Sutton, and James C. Bezdek. "Breast cancer detection using image processing techniques." *Ninth IEEE International Conference on Fuzzy Systems. FUZZ-IEEE 2000 (Cat. No. 00CH37063).* Vol. 2. IEEE, San Antonio, TX, USA, 2000.
29. Gupta, Siddhartha, et al. "Breast cancer detection using image processing techniques." *2019 Innovations in Power and Advanced Computing Technologies (i-PACT)*, Vol. 1. IEEE, Vellore, India, 2019.
30. Prakash, R. Meena, et al. "Segmentation of thermal infrared breast images using K-means, FCM and EM algorithms for breast cancer detection." *2017 International Conference on Innovations in Information, Embedded and Communication Systems (ICIIECS).* IEEE, Coimbatore, India, 2017.
31. Younis, Younis Samir, et al. "Early diagnosis of breast cancer using image processing techniques." *Journal of Nanomaterials* 2022 (2022): 1–6.
32. Varma, Chaitanya, and Omkar Sawant. "An alternative approach to detect breast cancer using digital image processing techniques." *2018 International Conference on Communication and Signal Processing (ICCSP).* IEEE (pp. 0134–0137), 2018.
33. Tomar, Ranjeet Singh, et al. "Analysis of breast cancer using image processing techniques." *2009 Third UKSim European Symposium on Computer Modeling and Simulation.* IEEE, Athens, Greece, 2009.
34. Sangeetha, R., and K. Srikanta Murthy. "A novel approach for detection of breast cancer at an early stage using digital image processing techniques." *2017 International Conference on Inventive Systems and Control (ICISC).* IEEE, 2017.
35. Alhadidi, Basim, Mohammad H. Zu'bi, and Hussam N. Suleiman. "Mammogram breast cancer image detection using image processing functions." *Information Technology Journal* 6.2 (2007): 217–221.
36. Moh'd Rasoul, A. Al-Hadidi, Mohammed Y. Al-Gawagzeh, and Bayan A. Alsaaidah. "Solving mammography problems of breast cancer detection using artificial neural networks and image processing techniques." *Indian Journal of Science and Technology* 5.4 (2012): 2520–2528.

37. Ramani, R., N. Suthanthira Vanitha, and S. Valarmathy. "The pre-processing techniques for breast cancer detection in mammography images." *International Journal of Image, Graphics and Signal Processing* 5.5 (2013): 47.
38. Tarique, Mohammed, et al. "Fourier transform based early detection of breast cancer by mammogram image processing." *Journal of Biomedical Engineering and Medical Imaging* 2.4 (2015): 17.
39. Singh, Anuj Kumar, and Bhupendra Gupta. "A novel approach for breast cancer detection and segmentation in a mammogram." *Procedia Computer Science* 54 (2015): 676–682.
40. Joro, R., et al. "Dynamic infrared imaging in identification of breast cancer tissue with combined image processing and frequency analysis." *Journal of Medical Engineering & Technology* 32.4 (2008): 325–335.
41. Helwan, Abdulkader, and Rahib H. Abiyev. "ISIBC: An intelligent system for identification of breast cancer." *2015 International Conference on Advances in Biomedical Engineering (ICABME)*. IEEE, Beirut, Lebanon, 2015.
42. Minavathi, S. Murali, and M. S. Dinesh. "Classification of mass in breast ultrasound images using image processing techniques." *International Journal of Computer Applications* 42.10 (2012): 29–36.
43. Charan, Saira, Muhammad Jaleed Khan, and Khurram Khurshid. "Breast cancer detection in mammograms using convolutional neural network." *2018 International Conference on Computing, Mathematics and Engineering Technologies (iCoMET)*. IEEE, Sukkur, Pakistan, 2018.
44. Tobore, Igbe, et al. "Deep learning intervention for health care challenges: Some biomedical domain considerations." *JMIR mHealth and uHealth* 7.8 (2019): e11966.
45. Altaf, Fouzia, et al. "Going deep in medical image analysis: Concepts, methods, challenges, and future directions." *IEEE Access* 7 (2019): 99540–99572.
46. Panayides, Andreas S., et al. "AI in medical imaging informatics: Current challenges and future directions." *IEEE Journal of Biomedical and Health Informatics* 24.7 (2020): 1837–1857.
47. Alber, Mark, et al. "Integrating machine learning and multiscale modeling—Perspectives, challenges, and opportunities in the biological, biomedical, and behavioral sciences." *NPJ Digital Medicine* 2.1 (2019): 115.
48. Attar, Hooyar, et al. "Additive manufacturing of low-cost porous titanium-based composites for biomedical applications: Advantages, challenges and opinion for future development." *Journal of Alloys and Compounds* 827 (2020): 154263
49. Younas, Zohaib, et al. "Mechanistic approaches to the application of nano-zinc in the poultry and biomedical industries: A comprehensive review of future perspectives and challenges." *Molecules* 28.3 (2023): 1064.
50. Grasso, Gerardo, Daniela Zane, and Roberto Dragone. "Microbial nanotechnology: Challenges and prospects for green biocatalytic synthesis of nanoscale materials for sensoristic and biomedical applications." *Nanomaterials* 10.1 (2019): 11.
51. Chan, Heang-Ping, Ravi K. Samala, and Lubomir M. Hadjiiski. "CAD and AI for breast cancer—Recent development and challenges." *The British Journal of Radiology* 93.1108 (2019): 20190580.
52. Aresta, Guilherme, et al. "Bach: Grand challenge on breast cancer histology images." *Medical Image Analysis* 56 (2019): 122–139.
53. Abdelhafiz, Dina, et al. "Deep convolutional neural networks for mammography: Advances, challenges and applications." *BMC Bioinformatics* 20 (2019): 1–20.
54. Bi, Wenya Linda, et al. "Artificial Intelligence in cancer imaging: Clinical challenges and applications." *CA: A Cancer Journal for Clinicians* 69.2 (2019): 127–157.
55. Ganvir, Neha N., and D. M. Yadav. "Filtering method for pre-processing mammogram images for breast cancer detection." *International Journal of Engineering and Advanced Technology* 9.1 (2019): 4222–4229.

56. He, Wenda, et al. "Breast image pre-processing for mammographic tissue segmentation." *Computers in Biology and Medicine* 67 (2015): 61–73.
57. Mina, Luqman Mahmood, and Nor Ashidi Mat Isa. "Preprocessing technique for mammographic images." *International Journal of Computer Science and Information Technology Research* 2.4 (2014): 226–231.
58. Beeravolu, Abhijith Reddy, et al. "Preprocessing of breast cancer images to create datasets for deep-CNN." *IEEE Access* 9 (2021): 33438–33463.
59. Kim, Hyeongseok, et al. "A novel pre-processing technique for improving image quality in digital breast tomosynthesis." *Medical Physics* 44.2 (2017): 417–425.
60. Bandyopadhyay, Samir Kumar. "Pre-processing of mammogram images." *International Journal of Engineering Science and Technology* 2.11 (2010): 6753–6758.
61. Sharma, Jaya, J. K. Rai, and R. P. Tewari. "Identification of pre-processing technique for enhancement of mammogram images." *2014 International Conference on Medical Imaging, m-Health and Emerging Communication Systems (MedCom)* (pp. 115–119). IEEE, 2014.
62. Ibrahim, Naglaa S. Ali, et al. "An algorithm for pre-processing and segmentation of mammogram images." *2016 11th International Conference on Computer Engineering & Systems (ICCES)*. IEEE, Cairo, Egypt, 2016.
63. Talha, Muhammad, Ghazali Bin Sulong, and Arfan Jaffar. "Preprocessing digital breast mammograms using adaptive weighted frost filter." *Biomedical Research* 27.4 (2016): 1407–1412.
64. Öztürk, Şaban, and Bayram Akdemir. "Effects of histopathological image pre-processing on convolutional neural networks." *Procedia Computer Science* 132 (2018): 396–403.
65. Sharma, Shubham, Archit Aggarwal, and Tanupriya Choudhury. "Breast cancer detection using machine learning algorithms." *2018 International Conference on Computational Techniques, Electronics, and Mechanical Systems (CTEMS)*. IEEE, Belgaum, India, 2018.
66. Bazazeh, Dana, and Raed Shubair. "Comparative study of machine learning algorithms for breast cancer detection and diagnosis." *2016 5th International Conference on Electronic Devices, Systems, and Applications (ICEDSA)*. IEEE, Ras Al Khaimah, United Arab Emirates, 2016.
67. Ak, Muhammet Fatih. "A comparative analysis of breast cancer detection and diagnosis using data visualization and machine learning applications." *Healthcare* 8.2 (2020): 111.
68. Vaka, Anji Reddy, Badal Soni, and Sudheer Reddy. "Breast cancer detection by leveraging Machine Learning." *ICT Express* 6.4 (2020): 320–324.
69. Alarabeyyat, Abdulsalam, and Mohannad Alhanahnah. "Breast cancer detection using k-nearest neighbor machine learning algorithm." *2016 9th International Conference on Developments in eSystems Engineering (DeSE)*. IEEE, Liverpool, UK, 2016.
70. Osareh, Alireza, and Bita Shadgar. "Machine learning techniques to diagnose breast cancer." *2010 5th International Symposium on Health Informatics and Bioinformatics*. IEEE, Liverpool, UK, 2010.
71. Nallamala, Sri Hari, Pragnyaban Mishra, and Suvarna Vani Koneru. "Breast cancer detection using machine learning way." *International Journal of Recent Technology and Engineering* 8.2–3 (2019): 1402–1405.
72. Omondiagbe, David A., Shanmugam Veeramani, and Amandeep S. Sidhu. "Machine learning classification techniques for breast cancer diagnosis." *IOP Conference Series: Materials Science and Engineering*. Vol. 495. IOP Publishing, 2019.
73. Tahmooresi, Maryam, et al. "Early detection of breast cancer using machine learning techniques." *Journal of Telecommunication, Electronic and Computer Engineering (JTEC)* 10.3-2 (2018): 21–27.

74. Bhise, Sweta, et al. "Breast cancer detection using machine learning techniques." *International Journal of Engineering Research & Technology* 10.7 (2021): 2278–0181.
75. Al Bataineh, Ali. "A comparative analysis of nonlinear machine learning algorithms for breast cancer detection." *International Journal of Machine Learning and Computing* 9.3 (2019): 248–254.
76. Dhahri, Habib, et al. "Automated breast cancer diagnosis based on machine learning algorithms." *Journal of Healthcare Engineering* 2019 (2019): 4253641.
77. Safdar, Sadia, et al. "Bio-imaging-based machine learning algorithm for breast cancer detection." *Diagnostics* 12.5 (2022): 1134.
78. Gbenga, Dada Emmanuel, et al. "Performance comparison of machine learning techniques for breast cancer detection." *Nova Journal of Engineering and Applied Sciences* 6.1 (2017): 1–8.
79. Shen, Li, et al. "Deep learning to improve breast cancer detection on screening mammography." *Scientific Reports* 9.1 (2019): 12495.
80. Mambou, Sebastien Jean, et al. "Breast cancer detection using infrared thermal imaging and a deep learning model." *Sensors* 18.9 (2018): 2799.
81. Ismail, Nur Syahmi, and Cheab Sovuthy. "Breast cancer detection based on deep learning technique." *2019 International UNIMAS STEM 12th engineering conference (EnCon)*. IEEE, Kuching, Malaysia, 2019.
82. Zheng, Jing, et al. "Deep learning assisted efficient AdaBoost algorithm for breast cancer detection and early diagnosis." *IEEE Access* 8 (2020): 96946–96954.
83. Das, Abhishek, et al. "Breast cancer detection using an ensemble deep learning method." *Biomedical Signal Processing and Control* 70 (2021): 103009.
84. Bai, Jun, et al. "Applying deep learning in digital breast tomosynthesis for automatic breast cancer detection: A review." *Medical Image Analysis* 71 (2021): 102049.
85. Sha, Zijun, Lin Hu, and Babak Daneshvar Rouyendegh. "Deep learning and optimization algorithms for automatic breast cancer detection." *International Journal of Imaging Systems and Technology* 30.2 (2020): 495–506.
86. Lotter, William, et al. "Robust breast cancer detection in mammography and digital breast tomosynthesis using an annotation-efficient deep learning approach." *Nature Medicine* 27.2 (2021): 244–249.
87. Khuriwal, Naresh, and Nidhi Mishra. "Breast cancer detection from histopathological images using deep learning." *2018 3rd International Conference and Workshops on Recent Advances and Innovations in Engineering (ICRAIE)*. IEEE, Jaipur, India, 2018.
88. Salvi, Siddhant, and Ameya Kadam. "Breast cancer detection using deep learning and IoT technologies." *Journal of Physics: Conference Series*. 1831 (2021): 012030.
89. Rashed, Essam, and M. Samir Abou El Seoud. "Deep learning approach for breast cancer diagnosis." *Proceedings of the 8th International Conference on Software and Information Engineering* (pp. 159–186), 2019.
90. Selvathi, D., and A. Aarthy Poornila. "Deep learning techniques for breast cancer detection using medical image analysis." In Jude Hemanth, Valentina Emilia Balas (eds). *Biologically Rationalized Computing Techniques for Image Processing Applications*, pp. 159–186, 2018.
91. Wang, Dayong, et al. "Deep learning for identifying metastatic breast cancer." *arXiv preprint arXiv:1606.05718* (2016).
92. Khuriwal, Naresh, and Nidhi Mishra. "Breast cancer diagnosis using deep learning algorithm." *2018 International Conference on Advances in Computing, Communication Control and Networking (ICACCCN)*. IEEE, Greater Noida, India, 2018.
93. Ragab, Dina A., et al. "Breast cancer detection using deep convolutional neural networks and support vector machines." *PeerJ* 7 (2019): e6201.
94. Khan, SanaUllah, et al. "A novel deep learning based framework for the detection and classification of breast cancer using transfer learning." *Pattern Recognition Letters* 125 (2019): 1–6.

95. Saber, Abeer, et al. "A novel deep-learning model for automatic detection and classification of breast cancer using the transfer-learning technique." *IEEE Access* 9 (2021): 71194–71209.
96. Sadoughi, Farahnaz, et al. "Artificial Intelligence methods for the diagnosis of breast cancer by image processing: A review." *Breast Cancer: Targets and Therapy* 10 (2018): 219–230.
97. Zheng, Dan, Xiujing He, and Jing Jing. "Overview of Artificial Intelligence in breast cancer medical imaging." *Journal of Clinical Medicine* 12.2 (2023): 419.
98. Mendes, João, et al. "AI in breast cancer imaging: A survey of different applications." *Journal of Imaging* 8.9 (2022): 228.
99. Hu, Qiyuan, and Maryellen L. Giger. "Clinical Artificial Intelligence applications: Breast imaging." *Radiologic Clinics* 59.6 (2021): 1027–1043.
100. Wang, Yang, et al. "Application of Artificial Intelligence based on deep learning in breast cancer screening and imaging diagnosis." *Neural Computing and Applications* 33 (2021): 9637–9647.
101. Lei, Yu-Meng, et al. "Artificial Intelligence in medical imaging of the breast." *Frontiers in Oncology* 11 (2021): 600557.
102. Le, E. P. V., Y. Wang, Yuan Huang, Sarah Hickman, and F. J. Gilbert "Artificial Intelligence in breast imaging." *Clinical radiology* 74.5 (2019): 357–366.
103. Tran, William T., et al. "Computational radiology in breast cancer screening and diagnosis using Artificial Intelligence." *Canadian Association of Radiologists Journal* 72.1 (2021): 98–108.
104. Sheth, Deepa, and Maryellen L. Giger. "Artificial Intelligence in the interpretation of breast cancer on MRI." *Journal of Magnetic Resonance Imaging* 51.5 (2020): 1310–1324.
105. Giordano, Chris, et al. "Accessing Artificial Intelligence for clinical decision-making." *Frontiers in Digital Health* 3 (2021): 645232.
106. Striani, Manuel, et al. "Artificial Intelligence in clinical decision support: A focused literature survey." *Yearbook of Medical Informatics* 28.01 (2019): 120–127.
107. Bennett, Casey C., and Kris Hauser. "Artificial Intelligence framework for simulating clinical decision-making: A Markov decision process approach." *Artificial Intelligence in Medicine* 57.1 (2013): 9–19.
108. Harish, Vinyas, et al. "Artificial Intelligence and clinical decision making: The new nature of medical uncertainty." *Academic Medicine* 96.1 (2021): 31–36.
109. Pedersen, Mangor, et al. "Artificial Intelligence for clinical decision support in neurology." *Brain Communications* 2.2 (2020): fcaa096.
110. Romero-Brufau, Santiago, et al. "A lesson in implementation: A pre-post study of providers' experience with Artificial Intelligence-based clinical decision support." *International Journal of Medical Informatics* 137 (2020): 104072.
111. Buchlak, Quinlan D., et al. "Machine learning applications to clinical decision support in neurosurgery: An Artificial Intelligence augmented systematic review." *Neurosurgical Review* 43 (2020): 1235–1253.
112. Hassan, Nehal, et al. "Preventing sepsis; how can Artificial Intelligence inform the clinical decision-making process? A systematic review." *International Journal of Medical Informatics* 150 (2021): 104457.
113. Bizzo, Bernardo C., et al. "Artificial Intelligence and clinical decision support for radiologists and referring providers." *Journal of the American College of Radiology* 16.9 (2019): 1351–1356.
114. Aljaaf, Ahmed J., et al. "Toward an optimal use of Artificial Intelligence techniques within a clinical decision support system." *2015 Science and Information Conference (SAI)*. IEEE, London, UK, 2015.

115. Sadoughi, Farahnaz, and Abbas Sheikhtaheri. "Applications of Artificial Intelligence in clinical decision making: Opportunities and challenges." *Health Information Management* 8.3 (2011): 353.
116. Yeo, Melissa, et al. "Artificial Intelligence in clinical decision support and outcome prediction—Applications in stroke." *Journal of Medical Imaging and Radiation Oncology* 65.5 (2021): 518–528.
117. Wu, Miao, et al. "Artificial Intelligence for clinical decision support in sepsis." *Frontiers in Medicine* 8 (2021): 665464.
118. Smith, Helen, and Kit Fotheringham. "Artificial Intelligence in clinical decision-making: Rethinking liability." *Medical Law International* 20.2 (2020): 131–154.
119. Loftus, Tyler J., et al. "Artificial Intelligence and surgical decision-making." *JAMA Surgery* 155.2 (2020): 148–158.

9 Cognitive Machine Learning-Based Intrusion Detection System for Identification of Life-Threatening Diseases

Sadaf Hussain, Tanweer Sohail, and Muhammad Adnan Khan

9.1 INTRODUCTION

The sooner someone is diagnosed, the better their outlook. The earlier we can detect diseases the more success that healthcare professionals will have in intervening with those treatment plans. This well-timed intervention leads to large improvements in patient outcomes in both survival and quality of life [1,2]. Cancer is one such example—early detection means better treatment and more opportunities to enter remission. Likewise, early detection of CVDs can enable therapeutic lifestyle changes and medications to prevent heart attacks and strokes [2,3].

This chapter focuses on how CML could be a game-changer for ascertaining the disease. In this paper, we introduce a unique radiological approach that can detect life-threatening medical conditions; this approach is called CML-based IDS (intrusion detection system). We will delve into CML and its subfields to provide a perspective into the functionality of processing the intricate web of medical data coming from a plethora of sources that include images, electronic health records, and biosensor data. This IDS built over CML, which incorporates deep learning for image analysis, natural language processing on text data, and reasoning capabilities would be able to detect subtle anomalies suggestive of a disease.

9.1.1 Escalating Burden of Life-Threatening Diseases

Most chronic diseases such as cancer, cardiovascular diseases, and neurological disorders are a major cause of worldwide over 70% of deaths [4]. Several works have suggested novel methods to tackle this important issue such as using IoT and ML technologies for early detection and managing chronic diseases [5]. This includes the hybrid optimization algorithm between Gravitational Search with Particle Swarm Optimization, which worked well to improve the specificity and sensitivity of

 DOI: 10.1201/9781003469896-9

classifiers for chronic kidney disease (CKD) and cardiovascular disease (CVD) [6]. In addition, a recent report proposed an inexpensive model of prediction scores based on routine blood tests for the long-term prognosis of various chronic disorders with high specificity, a precise means for recognizing the indices of chronic disease identification and clustering [7]. These advances are a testament to the acute demand for superior diagnostic approaches to deal with chronic diseases more effectively and drastically decrease the mortality rates attached to the ailments as well, echoing the WHO call to be stern about tackling the critical, worldwide health problem.

Discovering disease at an early stage is key to saving the lives of patients and cutting down on the number of deaths. The earlier an illness is detected, the better chance we have as healthcare providers to intervene with plans that we more confidently expect will succeed. The key to survival - and quality of life - is early intervention. The sooner cancer is identified, the more likely it is to respond to successful treatments and send your invitation to remission. In the same manner, diagnosing cardiovascular diseases in their early stage enables the application of lifestyle changes and drug therapy that may avert fatal conditions like heart attacks and strokes.

The pursuit to detect diseases such as Alzheimer's, diabetes, and dementia in their early stages has paved the way for the quest to find novel diagnostic tools which could be quick, accurate, and less invasive [8–11]. Looking into the future, CML is poised to change the way diseases are detected turning out to possibly be of great impact if healthcare principles are revamped in the process. As mentioned extrinsically, science has established that fibrillation risks can be predicted with a 96% detection rate in cases of dementia [11] tells us that machine learning algorithms can also get very high accuracies when it comes to predicting diseases similar to light diabetes. The result is not only improvement in early detection but also in personalized and high-efficacy healthcare interventions, resulting in patient outcomes and quality of life. In summary, the inclusion of CML into disease detection is a major milestone in the proactive and efficacious healthcare discipline.

9.1.2 Limitations of Traditional Diagnostics

The troubles with traditional diagnostic methods in healthcare traditional diagnostic methods in healthcare have major limitations that can thwart early and accurate disease detection, which in turn can affect patient outcomes. These inadequacies include a low detection rate, a delay in providing results, a low degree of automation, high cost, large-sized devices, and demand for professionals in central laboratory settings [12–14]. In addition, extensive use of centralized laboratory tests limited the testing capacity, in turn resulting in delays in the diagnosis as seen in infectious diseases, such as COVID-19 [15]. In response to these challenges, testing technologies are constantly being scaled down to eventually provide accurate, rapid, and portable testing at the point of care (POCTs), with the ability to test a much larger array of diseases [16].

Conventional incremental diagnostic approaches, such as the one based on tissue biopsy, more often than not result in significant delays in the prompt diagnosis and treatment initiation, particularly in the case of aggressive cancer types. Histopathology, the primary mode for cancer cell assessment according to research, is not real-time [17]. Alternatively, novel strategies such as telemedicine, asynchronous evaluation, and patient-led self-sampling devices have been shown to be convenient approaches for decreasing diagnostic delays in disorders like Axial Spondyloarthritis (axSpA) [18]. Another example includes studies among patients with inflammatory rheumatic diseases (IRD) which highlight the need for early triage and fast-track appointments to ensure timely commencement of treatment [19]. Moreover, the introduction of rapid diagnostic clinics, such as the Rapid Access Prostate Imaging and Diagnosis (RAPID) pathway has demonstrated an improvement in the diagnostic times for prostate cancer [20]. A similar acceleration of diagnosis has been in the field of pulmonary medicine with mediastinal and hilar lesions using endobronchial ultrasound-guided transbronchial needle aspiration (EBUS-TBNA), minimizing delays in treatment initiation [21].

Similarly, analyzing medical data (X-rays, blood tests) is fundamentally manual and, therefore, potentially subjective, and can suffer from fatigue, we know that humans only have limited information processing abilities, so they are prone to the possibility of both false negatives and false positives when a diagnosis is missed or misinterpreted. The application of artificial in of artificial intelligence (AI) and deep-learning algorithms is another strategy that eLearning authors are utilizing to automate error discovery within medical datasets, which has demonstrably improved overall accuracy and efficiency [22]. Advanced AI such as the BERT model is used for top-level clinical note analysis with the prediction of morbidities in the future, which removes the load of human experts, and the output quality improved [23]. Finally, we also developed a novel method called Untrainable Data Cleansing that provides for the automated detection of low-quality data for maintaining patient privacy and to enhance the generalizability of AI while reducing the cost of training and time, all around assuring fair evaluation of AI performance [24]. Trained with already existing algorithms for various purposes, it uses automation, standardization, advanced imaging, molecular techniques, and data analytics, to mention but a few, to improve the quality, reliability as well as the efficiency of medical analysis [25].

Colonoscopies or exploratory surgery can be part of the diagnosis process; however, they can be invasive procedures that cause discomfort and potential complications for the patient, and the need for adopting this framework for the diagnosis leads to many patients avoiding the exams and diagnostic tests that may be important for their health. Naeem et al. [26] demonstrated that adverse events associated with bowel preparation for colonoscopy, such as vomiting, epistaxis, and abdominal pain. The completion rate of colonoscopy by general surgeons has also been found to be about 49.1%, with reasons for failure including inadequate bowel preparation and intolerant patients [27]. Research on the complications related to invasive diagnostic procedures after screening for lung cancer showed a median excess complication rate of 16.6 per 1,000, identifying that following screening for lung cancer, adherence to clinical guidelines is important to avoid avoidable harm [28]. For the pain of colonoscopy, viewing real-time videos of the procedure has been reported to reduce pain and anxiety and enhance satisfaction with a high compliance ratio [29].

The above limitations related to virus-specific techniques reflect a great necessity for novel diagnostic tools that can address these issues. While the remaining sections of this blog develop further on CML, it will now be logical to hope that we can use it to rather provide faster, more accurate, and less invasive ways of getting to know who is truly sick with a life-threatening disease.

9.1.3 Cognitive Machine Learning: A Paradigm Shift

CML, a new form of artificial intelligence, constitutes a departure from the traditional methods of diagnostics to help identify diseases in healthcare. CML is a field that has been designed to combine multiple traditional machine learning methods together, and also activating many subfields from AI in order to mimic human cognitive processes to make a more versatile system to analyze complex medical data and detect patterns that may not be seen by human eye. In this way, CML, among the highlights, is the diagnosis of cancer, hitherto there have been many advances in the field of oncology; it is a revolution in the treatment of blood cancers like chronic myeloid leukemia. Machine learning (ML) algorithms have demonstrated the capacity to classify CML subtypes here, more notably when integrating biochemical, biomolecular, imaging, and clinical data as well as to forecast disease progression and evaluate treatment response [30,31]. Such algorithms contribute a helpful instrument to mechanically examine the diagnosis of CML by dealing with the image processing of stained blood microscope photos, thus improving the reliability and efficiency of leukemia screening [32]. In addition, deployment of ML models in CML patients could prove to be a powerful tool for risk stratification, therapeutic decision-making and ultimately, disease control in the rapidly changing approach toward overall management of CML [2].

The powerful performance of deep learning algorithms, especially Convolutional Neural Networks (CNNs), in interpreting various imaging modalities, including X-rays, CT scans, and MRIs, has revolutionized medical image analysis [34–36]. CNNs are particularly skilled at finding very slight irregularities in the mountains of data that people produce - which can serve as early warnings of diseases - and can allow doctors to diagnose people better and sooner. Deep learning integration in healthcare systems is a breakthrough in the workings of image classification, object detection, and segmentation problems, which are seen to be a remedy for the present healthcare system hectic battles. Nevertheless, the scarcity of large-scale medical datasets continues to be a crucial obstacle that affects the generalization and performance of deep learning models in medical image analysis.

Common NLP applications in healthcare include NLP analysis of doctor's notes, lab reports, and discharge summaries, which is critical for extracting useful information from unstructured text data and enables Clinical Decision Support Systems to be leveraged for effective processing of information [37,38]. These reports are analyzed with NLP methods (classification, prediction, Word Sense Disambiguation, Segmentation, and word Embedding) to extract important details like risk factors, disease mentions, medication interactions, etc., that can be useful for disease identification and in improving the patient care [39]. Systematically converted unstructured clinical texts into structured formats by NLP models and made unstructured clinical texts converted into unstructured formats to be mined into detailed clinical information in specific clinical study areas for applications in clinical research, trial design, and safety assessments of regulatory submissions using Real-World Data (RWD) [40].

Cognitive machine learning (CML) provides the tools needed to embed reasoning into healthcare systems with the goal of making decisions in an informed manner using previous medical knowledge and a large range of data sources [31,41]. For example, an X-ray can analyze much better when combined with a patient history along with lab results, and a CML system can be used to do the same [41]. This holistic method helps in significantly increasing the level of diagnostic accuracy and allows the system to compute the impact of interventions and hence supports making clinical decisions actionable [42]. In the study of chronic myeloid leukemia and multiple myeloma, very patient-centric approaches have been advocated that focus on the behavioral, psychosocial, and interactional parts of care as paramount to care and patient outcomes [43].

9.2 INTRUSION DETECTION SYSTEMS (IDS) IN HEALTHCARE

The area of healthcare data analysis approach to traditional IDS can be implemented using CML to find out patterns that indicate towards life-threatening diseases by being able to trace displeasing behavior of physiological states. Using several forms of data, including medical images like X-ray CT scans and MRIs, a CML-based IDS is capable of identifying such things as tumors or lesions, therefore helping the IDS to detect disease at an early stage. This system may integrate information from various sources such as patient's medical records, positive findings on investigations, and laboratory results to improve the diagnostic capabilities of a clinical assessment as well as provide a holistic picture of a patient's state [44]. With the prognosis and machine learning algorithms added to it, the system can comprehend the healthcare data and explore possible health dangers to build the patient's quality of life.

In this study, Contextually Enhanced Electronic Health Records (EHRs) become handy in providing the IDS with an extensive database containing patients' medical profiles and profile identifiers, such as past medical history, prescribed medications, and test results to check for emerging health issues based on trends and variability. Biosensors can be integrated into clothes and shoes to monitor individuals' health parameters in real time, and the IDS can notice changes, which indicate the development of a new illness [45]. Wanting this strong and heterogeneous data continually processed, a cognitive IDS based on machine learning can accurately detect less conspicuous outliers, which may signify the onset of potentially lethal states and require further examination for timely treatment [45]. In combination with biosensors, the IDS serves as a smart loom, aided by EHRs, to support continuous healthcare surveillance thus promoting patient welfare through monitoring and early detection of diseases.

9.2.1 Redefining Intrusion for Healthcare

Within the frame of healthcare exposure, the IDS concept transforms into a vital health guardian mend anticipation scanning numerous outlets of the different types of data to identify what differs from the standard patterns of the healthy condition and may be compared to the security guard for health. This is even similar to the proposed subclass IDS for healthcare known as the Intrusion Detection System for the Internet of Healthcare Things [46]. Where IDS tries to identify the anomalies that could signify the presence of severe diseases just like an IDS tries to identify threats in computer networks. Therefore, the security threats of the Internet of Everything (IoE), particularly in the healthcare sector, create prominent challenges for dealing with the tremendous volume of medical information, which cannot be effectively managed without high-level IDS algorithms such as the Artificial Immune System (AIS) based IDS. As pattern recognition and machine learning strategy, IDS in healthcare becomes capable of detecting the indicated anomalous pattern in patients' data and providing appropriate alerts before the life-threatening factors emerge.

IDS in healthcare, through pattern recognition and machine learning, can effectively determine complex high-risk patterns in patient data for timely intervention for adverse health outcomes that may lead to life-threatening ailments. Intrusion Detection System (IDS) to monitor patient health data continuously in healthcare, as discussed in the various research papers [47,48], can function effectively as a method for discovering possible anomalies and is considered an important for early detection and more proactive healthcare. Drawing and maintaining a continual reference to a baseline of a patient's vital statistics, as well as other input from another source such as wearables and diagnostic procedures, a CML-based IDS can quickly discern patterns that indicate a potential health event such as a sudden increase in blood pressure or irregular findings in scans. This action plan enhances the identification of critical illnesses in their initial stages due to increased rates of evaluation and hence improves the likelihood of patient outcomes in alarming diseases.

9.2.2 Data Sources for IDS in Healthcare

While General Machine Learning (GML) in IDS as a tool is considerably useful, CML in IDS does have the unique capability to leverage a plethora of data types for improved anomaly detection. These enable the IDS to accumulate information from disparate sources, including medical images like X-rays CT scans, and MRI to pinpoint less obvious anomalies that signify highly pathological health conditions. These procedures involve usual X-ray or CT scan images, which are saved in the CML system; the deep learning algorithms help in analyzing these images that can detect fractures, tumors or any type of human body distortions with high efficiency. This approach not only performs an alert for further investigation but also enables early diagnosis, showing the valuable starting of using rich data sources in IDS for better detection and decisions [46,49].

Electronic Health Records (EHRs) is a centralized information system of a patient's medical information, which includes a list of diagnoses, medications, allergies, and laboratory results, which allow the IDS to analyze numerous records at once and identify trends or potentially malicious activities [45]. Furthermore, when embedded with rich patient data from EHRs, such as abrupt changes in the red blood cell count or blood glucose level along with genetic preconditions like diabetes and antigens, the IDS can notify healthcare providers about the potential development of an illness and facilitate early interventions in chronic diseases. The proactive approach demonstrated through data mining of EHR presents the concepts of early identification as not only a viable strategy but also as a valuable method of optimizing patient outcomes and the general workings of healthcare systems [38].

Smart wearables are the key technology that is able to keep track of various parameters of a patient's health, ranging from the regularly measured vital signs to other physiological markers, all in real time [50]. Smart devices are described as having high innovation, accurate sensing of the body, and wireless connection that brings comfort in health measurement for individual use [51]. Further, wearable chemical sensors allow for biomarker discovery from other less invasive body fluids constantly using the human body as the sample; this can culminate in biomarker discovery for precision medicine [52]. The next generation of wearables will focus more on biochemical sensing with secretions and excreted liquids such as sweat and interstitial fluids, expanding the realm of health status assessment and early disease diagnosis. An IDS contains several sources of information and uses the CML networks to analyze this endless stream of information; this means that it is possible to diagnose the health status of a specific body part to detect any signs of abnormality which will in turn improve the well-being of human beings as new mechanisms for diagnosing diseases are developed to encourage a faster approach to diseases that affect certain body organs.

9.2.3 Cognitive Machine Learning for Disease Identification

CML stands for CML, which is an enabling concept of disease identification by applying different branches of artificial intelligence as described in the papers [53]. The operational theoretic constituents empower CML to provide optimal performance in attempting various medical-related data types such as medical images, EHRs, and biosensor data from wearable devices [54]. The machine learning algorithms adopted in CML, such as the Convolutional Neural Networks (CNNs), possess high accuracy as pertains to image recognition and thus are able to differentiate sample images with such minuteness that may not be easily distinguishable even by human eyes. By integrating these future-oriented technologies, CML has the capability to supplement disease detection by identifying diseases at an early stage through the usage of new technologies with improved accuracy without the drawbacks conventional diagnostic tests present.

The help of NLP is crucial when it comes to acquiring knowledge from unarranged medical textual data like doctors' notes and reports by filtering the most important data like the risks that are involved, the diseases that may be associated, and medication interactions, among others [55]. With the help of NLP algorithms, prescient and specific clinical details that may be imprecise or missing can be formalized and added to structured datasets, thereby improving the General clinical understanding that the CML system has of a patient's condition. Through changing the text data into more manageable formats, NLP is able to help to detect diseases at an earlier stage and also to enhance the methods used in clinical research, trials, and safety assessments, and therefore to assist in the ultimate goal of providing the high level of patient care and the better decision-making in the medical field [40].

CML goes beyond ML by integrating cognitive reasoning capabilities as presented in several academic papers [56–58]. The CML system can use the blood test of a patient, the patient's medical history records, and a recent X-ray to improve its outlook on potential diseases, thus improving the overall degree of accuracy in the disease diagnosis. Indeed, integrating reason occurring in medical reasoning with prior medical knowledge and other data inputs prepares healthcare professionals with a comprehensive diagnostic tool, even for chronic conditions, which ideally translates to the betterment of patient outcomes in the long run. If combined from data of different modalities obtained from patients or clinical practices, an outcome such as that observed in CML can highlight the potential for such a tool to change healthcare by allowing for more accurate and timely interventions based on fully instantiated, data- and reason-driven data analysis and data reasoning.

9.3 UNLOCKING THE POWER OF CML

CML is a blend of multiple subfields of artificial intelligence that has transformed the identification of diseases as found in the research materials. Due to many merits for medical analysis, including accelerated results, increased precision, and being minimally invasive, the application of CML addresses the shortcomings of conventional diagnostics [53,54,59]. CML; fusing the hi-tech engineering hardware with AI and ML, infers the occurrence of chronic diseases, including heart issues, brain tumors, and diabetes; in disease forecasting, the successes are demonstrative. Also, the facet of cognitive science of the diagnostic process is that cognitive bias, as well as the improvements in decision-making calibration, should be incorporated into medical training, asserting the medical trainees' demand for the cognition of cognitive science concepts that would contribute to the formation of clinical reasoning and decision-making acumen [60]. Due to this blend of approaches, scholars are identifying all types of life-threatening diseases well in advance and this step changes the method of identifying diseases and it is one of the contributions of CML from the subfields of AI.

9.3.1 Deep Learning

Convolutional Neural Networks (CNNs) have emerged as highly efficient in medical image analysis as seen in deep learning algorithms. By training the CNN on large volumetric medical imaging such as X-ray images, CT, and MRI, the CNN can identify anomalies that would be most likely otherwise overlooked by human eyes [61]. For instance, one can envision an actual CNN, developed as an outline of millions of mammograms; it would be presumably accurate in identifying early signs of breast cancer to allow for better outcomes through earlier intervention [62]. In addition, CNNs that are trained in the context of retinal scans can diagnose diabetic retinopathy, a complication associated with diabetes that can lead to blindness. 'A' Because of the advanced identification of DR using CNN, treatments are given beforehand to avoid the progression of DR, demonstrating the effectiveness of CNNs in almost all diseases [36].

9.3.2 Natural Language Processing (NLP)

Although Natural Language Processing (NLP) is used to handle unstructured medical data like doctor's notes and discharge summaries, it is helpful to improve the effectiveness of CML (ML) systems that require such data [37,39]. NLP algorithms can pinpoint the risk factors because the data contains significant words that refer to the patient's vulnerability to a particular disease, such as appearing on the screen phrases that signal a family history of cardiovascular diseases in the patient's electronic record, which will be appreciated by Cognitive ML system and help improve the decision-making process [63]. Thus, through NLP approaches, healthcare professionals can rapidly analyze large volumes of unprocessed text information, enhancing patients' care, contributing to explorative clinical research, and thus pointing to at-risk patients and their vulnerability to specific diseases, further aiming to increase the effectiveness of treatments and the quality of provided healthcare services.

At this juncture, it is paramount to take a look at how Natural Language Processing (NLP) is important in combating challenges in the healthcare sector through extracting disease mentions and medication interactions from the unstructured text data as evidenced in the following papers. NLP methods were used to diagnose health issues from social media feeds clearly [64], discharge actionable details from pharmacovigilance texts for drug safety [65], and build frameworks for the extraction of medication details from clinical texts to help decipher drug changes [66]. Furthermore, NLP applications can delineate people with dementia medication mentions and analyze the usage of medication compared to records of primary care [55]. Furthermore, when it is coupled with text mining, NLP can extract drug-drug interactions from text, aiding clinicians in prescription choices improving the Cognitive ML system's awareness of a patient's health status, and enabling the detection of diseases and preventing adverse drug reactions before occurrence [67].

9.3.3 Reasoning Capabilities

CML (ML) systems, empowered by deep learning and natural language processing (NLP) [59], play a pivotal role in revolutionizing disease identification by integrating reasoning capabilities. By analyzing a patient's medical history, blood test results, and X-ray images collectively, Cognitive ML systems can make more informed decisions about potential diseases, significantly enhancing accuracy [60]. This approach aligns with the need for improved clinical reasoning and decision-making in healthcare, as highlighted in cognitive science research [48]. Moreover, the application of cognitive reasoning tools has shown a small but clinically important improvement in diagnostic accuracy for medical professionals and students, emphasizing the practical impact of such systems in real-world settings [56]. By leveraging these advanced technologies, Cognitive ML acts as a powerful ally in the early and accurate identification of life-threatening diseases, ultimately leading to enhanced patient outcomes and improved healthcare services.

9.4 COGNITIVE ML-BASED INTRUSION DETECTION SYSTEM ARCHITECTURE

Using insights from Cognitive ML, IDS systems transform from defending computer networks to safeguarding human health in the field of healthcare data security [49]. Cognitive ML, which is a combination of AI subfields, helps in processing complex medical data forms such as medical images, electronic health records, and biosensor data [68]. Thus, through deep learning for image analysis, natural language processing for text data, and reasoning capabilities, Cognitive ML-based IDS systems are capable of interpreting this abundance of diverse data [69]. This transformation improves the capacity of the system to identify and alert malicious activities in health sectors, safeguard sensitive patient data as well as applied advanced AI features for a powerful and efficient analysis of all the acquired data.

9.4.1 Data Pre-Processing

The absence of data poses a challenge to CML (ML) models striving to deliver accurate statistical estimations and diagnostic evidence in academic achievement contexts [70]. There are older and often used methods for dealing with missing data in ML known as feature imputation and label prediction, which, to work, require assumptions about data distributions, which brings bias into the process. However, new approaches by researchers suggest other promising approaches, such as the CL frameworks where observed data with missing values do not need to be imputed and which has been shown to improve the performance and interpretability of ML [71]. Also, the fair ML is closely related to the topic as the authors note that missing data, if not dealt with properly, makes the situation worse and has a negative impact on both the accuracy and fairness in the classifications of nodes in the given graph [70]. Overall, missing data issues in ML are significant, and when properly handled, they can significantly enhance predictions while minimizing biased parameter estimation.

The features of clean and standardized data are helpful in improving the efficiency of Cognitive ML algorithms in treating the students in healthcare domain. Thus, by using Cognitive ML algorithms and ensuring the cleanliness and standardization of data, Cognitive Systems can start understanding the patterns present in the prepared data sets, which in turn allows for better recognition of anomalies and consequently, the improvement of disease diagnosing skills [59]. It may also be important to perform rigorous data cleansing prior to extracting features since lack of consistency and missing values affects the successful extraction of features necessary in the identification of disease patterns by the system [72]. Accurate anomaly detection enhances reliable decision-making in the healthcare of patients by getting the Intrusion Detection Systems (IDS) enhanced using Cognitive ML to provide healthcare experts with reliable health insights as preferred by the system [73]. Thus, pre-processing steps, including proper cleaning, formatting, and standardization of health care data are some of the important and basic requirements to support increased utilization of Cognitive ML-based IDS with the potential for better early diagnosis of severe diseases.

9.4.2 Feature Extraction Using Cognitive ML Techniques

Cognitive ML applies advanced deep learning algorithms, including the CNNs [74,75], to extract the right features from screens such as the X rays, CT scans, and MRIs. Particularly, although a CNN operates on a volumetric input in the given context of a breast cancer detection, a model trained on a rich database of mammograms is capable of detecting such essential characteristics as breast tissue density, ensembles of microstructures, and uneven masses, thus being efficient in early-stage breast cancer identification with high accuracy [75]. Secondly, NLP approaches help to obtain clinical information from Electronic Healthcare records for better management decision support, patient care optimization, and drug discovery through pattern analysis [76]. In addition, the use of Generative Adversarial Networks (GANs) as methods in oncological medical event extraction data augmentation for improving transfer learning of the model is described [77]. Artificial intelligence and more particularly, deep learning technologies are crucial in designing new models as they help discover latent features in the data feeds prevalent in the healthcare sector to identify diseases efficiently.

Deep learning techniques, such as Convolutional Neural Networks (CNNs), are not only valuable for cancer detection but also extend to identifying diabetic retinopathy from retinal scans by extracting features related to blood vessel abnormalities [39]. Moreover, Natural Language Processing (NLP) plays a crucial role in processing unstructured medical text data, enabling CML (ML) systems to extract essential features. Preventive NLP screening can include disease risk, family illness, heart, specific symptoms, and drug-drug interactions that would enable the identification of such cases and hence reduce the incidence of ADRs [66,78]. The convergence of deep learning and NLP presented here can be seen as an example of how increased cognitive healthcare is another method with real potential to improve decision-making and patient triaging.

By providing such informative features from the text, the Cognitive ML system broadens its accession to a patient's health condition. In combination, this allows a holistic picture and enables one to look for disease signatures or other unexpected patterns within the unstructured text, increasing the chances of disease detection. By utilizing the Cognitive ML framework, specific deep learning as a part of NLP, performs powerful feature extraction. It begets the hidden combinations that hide in different health data and ensures the correct identification of diseases and, therefore, the outcomes of patients.

9.4.3 Anomaly Detection

There are two main approaches systems use to identify deviations from normal patterns in extracted features that could indicate a life-threatening disease:

9.4.3.1 Statistical Techniques

Standardizing what is considered normal in Characteristics is one way, how it performs, especially in statistics as used in bioinformatics and medical studies. This can be achieved using methods such as the thresholds method or the Z scores. The thresholds include setting a limit to each individual characteristic with the aid of deviation from the average within a particular population, whereby any value that is beyond this limit is considered anomalous [4,26]. On the other hand, Z scores indicate how many standard units away from the expected value a particular score is with higher Z scores denoting abnormal scores. These techniques are intended for zeroing upon the data values and discrepancies of the pattern if the input data involved large populations of normal health individual data or specific patient data in retrospect for analysis. They serve as aids in reaching decisions and conclusions where research and data analysis are the main activities.

9.4.3.2 Machine Learning Techniques

Critical importance is anomaly detection in machine learning algorithms, and the clustering and classification algorithms on which it relies. These are trained on labeled datasets and used to identify such patterns in other unseen data through precise relationships between features [79]. In case of fatal diseases, such procedures can employ the attributes of medical scans, blood tests, or sensors to seek for symptoms that are early as those of ailments, such as cancer or heart problems [79]. Such systems, for instance, could identify disease states such as a human body lacking certain blood components or diagnosing new and unascertained ECG variances as potentially threatening [80]. However, using machinery learning methods for detecting anomalies in measurable variables can enhance the rate and quality of diagnosing diseases in healthcare facilities, thus improving patient's successes. Contrary to what it may imply, anomalies do not solely refer to life-threatening diseases. This can be due to other reasons like the use of substances and also could be a result of some health conditions that are transient.

Used most often as a first-line analysis pointing to potential issues that need further attention from a medical professional. For this purpose, the anomaly detection process is performed using such systems on extracted feature sets that may play an important role in identifying hidden diseases with prompt therapy and follow-up [80]. For instance, machines that contain sensors have saved many lives already by detecting anomalies indicative of fatal diseases at their early stages before it is too late. It uses various mathematical models, including artificial immune system (AIS), Self-Organized Maps(SOM), Min-Max Neural Networks (MMNN), Support Vector Machines(SVM), and Genetic Algorithms(GAs) that have been used as toolkits in classifying/segmenting clusters but none has been observed focusing on multiple diseases. Owing to its effectiveness when implemented within decision support systems (DSSs), Bayesian theory has also been used successfully for classification during the diagnosis stage before appropriate treatment is prescribed.

9.4.4 Decision-Making Module

The third and final part of the system concatenates the anomaly detection results and the rationale abilities that are associated with the final decision made; however, it should be noted that there are important limitations to the system. A good model combines anomaly scores on a variety of features, tests them statistically, and scores using z scores or probabilities from machine learning models [81]. These also incorporate patient details, such as patient history, demographics, current medications, prior anomaly reports, and additional suppressors, and are used to further refine the performances of the network for more accurate anomaly detection [82]. This sort of information provides the system with a more holistic view of a patient's history and current well-being, potentially resulting in a much finer-grain analysis of anomalies. As a result, this complete-process-oriented way of anomaly detection improves the overall anomaly detection process more robustly and makes it more useful with patient-specific details, other than its statistical anomaly detection aspect [83].

Rule-based systems are a new area of research in the field of reasoning and decision-making in healthcare with significant importance [60]. Rule-Based systems - Interpret anomaly scores and context that is combined with anomaly AND contextual information conform to predefined rules/ logics that can be (have to be)part of a criteria for alerting [60]. At a higher level, probabilistic reasoning with Bayesian networks can perform inference about the probability of disease presence given anomaly scores and contextual information, which can increase the significance of health diagnostic steps [84]. Health systems generate various outcomes depending on their integrated analysis results—no alert if low risk, information highlighting concerning features, critical alerts requiring immediate medical attention for possibly life-threatening conditions emphasizing the importance of effective alert generation and follow-up mechanisms in decision-making in healthcare [40].

When appropriate, we must also develop reasoning systems and algorithms that recognize these limitations and refrain from making unwarranted confident claims in the domain of anomaly detection in healthcare that frequents uncertainty and frequent incomplete medical data [85]. While some anomaly detection can be used for early disease detection, human judgment plays a critical role since providers leverage clinical knowledge and PCC-specific context to interpret alerts and make final diagnosis and treatment decisions [81]. Anomaly detection with reasoning potentially acts as a useful tool to alert healthcare professionals in a partnership where the system suggests issues to be considered further and depends on human judgment for the final decision, thus re-emphasizing the supportive nature of such systems in healthcare [86].

9.5 BENEFITS AND CHALLENGES OF COGNITIVE ML-BASED IDS

It is possible to increase the effectiveness of disease identification by using special intrusion detection systems designed for healthcare [87,88]. The mental advantages of utilizing Cognitive ML in this aspect are viewed as the ideal eradicating human constrains, for example, fatigue, inundation of information, and time constraints that may impede proper sickness diagnosis by doctors [48]. Likewise, CML models can parse large data sets such as MRIs, X-rays, and patient data, meaning that they afford full and fast data triage. However, it is rather unlikely that the manner in which CML accomplishes pattern recognition will not be as effective as that of human beings; in addition, CML is equipped with the ability to discern intricate relations or stream hitherto unnoticed people hence leading to rather accurate and earlier diagnoses particularly for complicated or rare diseases [59].

IDS can be updated by using machine learning for constant redevelopment, performance, and response, rapid enhancement in rate, easiness in scaling, and a decline in costs. Tan et al. [89] pointed out that by using large volumes of network traffic data, machine learning algorithms could be effectively used to classify intricate attack patterns. Cognitive IDS is a form of IDS that is fueled by machine learning algorithms capable of identifying menace in real time as well as analyzing, and mitigating them independently of human input. Also, due to the increasing occurrence of enterprises, there will be an increasing amount of data and its intensity that machine learning model must undergo to ensure an efficient detection as well as response towards threats, among other things. Hence purposely designed cognizant systems that can distinguish and respond to various forms of cyber threats in an organization can rather be developed [60].

The impact of delay is likely to have potentially harmful consequences on the outcome of individual's treatment. As the case may be with the diseases that pose these risks, these medical conditions should be diagnosed in their early stages [90]. Relating to the case of CML, the models make it possible to track different data streams in real time, making it easier to detect possible medical complications [91]. These models highlight the early developmental stages of diseases, relating to primary symptoms and showing how one may alter extracted features in data to alter possibilities for good therapeutic outcomes at an earlier stage than before positive symptoms develop. Thus, when integrating diverse datasets, machine learning methods have been proven to offer accurate classification that identifies the early stages of downhill cognitive dexterity that could still be arrested.

When CML is enhanced by data elements such as medical history, genetic predisposition, or personal behavior, individuals who are at high risk of contracting the virus can be easily identified enabling preventive action to be taken. This could, in turn, result in what has been referred to as precision medicine, which will have treatments that are outlined by individual characters and diseases. The implementation of CML-based IDS can bring about cost reduction by reducing unnecessary invasive procedures and avoiding complications arising from unnecessary practice in addition to the disproportionate designation of manpower effort to cases through accelerating IDS flow and allowing experienced staff to focus on challenging cases [48]. However, there are always hurdles, such as the ability to encourage patients and practitioners to take the right actions on given information so that CML can fit perfectly in the healthcare sector.

9.6 CONCLUSION

Various forms of diagnostics that are considered traditional, moreover, can have their specific drawbacks in terms of speed, accuracy, and the level of invasiveness. Cognitive ML (CML) is a game changer that affects the identification of diseases in amazing ways. As it has been viewed in this chapter, other elementary uses of this strategy encompass the subfields of this technique, including the deep learning technique, natural language processing capability, and capacity of reasoning. We talked about how crucial data preprocessing is as it is responsible for removing any off-quality data and normalizing the data for analysis. There is also an added value of showing how these techniques help in revealing hidden patterns essential in chronic diseases, mainly; Image analysis techniques in Deep Learning and text data extraction in NLP. Then, at the architectural level, we presented the Cognitive ML-based Intrusion Detection System proposed for healthcare data. This technology is a leap ahead because it uses Cognitive ML to identify diseases beyond any etiologic reasoning. Still, when applied with AI's enhanced ability, this method has the potential to revolutionize the healthcare system that is in place today and that potentially can utilize artificial intelligence (AI). Just imagine when medical experts will be able to input large doses of information into cognitive machine learning capable of winnowing the pile with medical images to blood test results, or doctor's notes, with a considerable level of accuracy to identify signs of a disease in patients' records if true, thereby could lead to better patient outcomes resulting from early detection of the diseases and enhanced treatment planning. However, it is crucial to note that data privacy, regulations, and AI explainability are still issues that we cannot overlook nonetheless, the benefits of Cognitive ML as a tool for disease identification cannot be overemphasized. Cognitive ML is a promising area of study in this field where it can act as a game-changer in the healthcare industry and consequent progress towards the concept of personalized medicine that will result in improved health standards for the human community.

REFERENCES

1. N. E. Almansouri et al., "Early Diagnosis of Cardiovascular Diseases in the Era of Artificial Intelligence: An In-Depth Review," *Cureus*, vol. 16, no. 3, Mar. 2024, doi: 10.7759/CUREUS.55869.
2. M. J. Oude Wolcherink, C. M. Behr, X. G. L. V. Pouwels, C. J. M. Doggen, and H. Koffijberg, "Health Economic Research Assessing the Value of Early Detection of Cardiovascular Disease: A Systematic Review," *Pharmacoeconomics*, vol. 41, no. 10, pp. 1183–1203, Oct. 2023, doi: 10.1007/S40273-023-01287-2.
3. "Early Detection and Prevention of Heart Disease I MyCardiologist." https://mycardiologist.net/early-detection-and-prevention-of-heart-disease/ (accessed June 07, 2024).
4. N. Nigar, A. Jaleel, S. Islam, M. K. Shahzad, and E. A. Affum, "IoMT Meets Machine Learning: From Edge to Cloud Chronic Diseases Diagnosis System," *J. Healthc. Eng.*, vol. 2023, pp. 1–13, Jun. 2023, doi: 10.1155/2023/9995292.
5. S. Kavi Priya and N. Saranya, "An Intelligent Approach for Accurate Prediction of Chronic Diseases," *Comput. Syst. Sci. Eng.*, vol. 46, no. 2, pp. 2571–2587, Jan. 2023, doi: 10.32604/CSSE.2023.031761.
6. J. Moini, O. Akinso, K. Ferdowsi, and M. Moini, "Chronic Diseases and Risks," *Heal. Care Today United States*, pp. 283–322, Jan. 2023, doi: 10.1016/B978-0-323-99038-7.00022-9.
7. M. Liu et al., "A Computational Framework of Routine Test Data for the Cost-Effective Chronic Disease Prediction," *Brief. Bioinform.*, vol. 24, no. 2, Feb. 2023, doi: 10.1093/BIB/BBAD054.
8. D. Barragán-Guerrero, M. Au, G. Gagnon, F. Gagnon, and P. Giard, "Early-Detection Scheme Based on Sequential Tests for Low-Latency Communications," *Eurasip J. Wirel. Commun. Netw.*, vol. 2023, no. 1, Mar. 2023, doi: 10.1186/S13638-023-02240-9.
9. E. Zhang, "Alzheimer's Disease: Why Is Early Detection Important?" *J. Student Res.*, vol. 12, no. 2, May 2023, doi: 10.47611/JSRHS.V12I2.4233.
10. A. H. Ataya, "Early Detection of Diabetes Using Machine Learning Techniques," *Proc. 3rd Int. Conf. Artif. Intell. Smart Energy, ICAIS 2023,* pp. 886–891, Feb. 2023, doi: 10.1109/ICAIS56108.2023.10073861.
11. M. S. Kabir, J. Khanom, M. A. Bhuiyan, Z. N. Tumpa, S. K. F. Rabby, and S. Bilgaiyan, "The Early Detection of Dementia Disease Using Machine Learning Approach," *2023 Int. Conf. Comput. Commun. Informatics, ICCCI 2023*, pp. 1–6, Jan. 2023, doi: 10.1109/ICCCI56745.2023.10128411.
12. J. Alzeer, J. Alzeer, and H. Benmerabet, "Recognizing Limitations: Overcoming Challenges in Enhancing Health and Preventing Disease," *Eur. J. Gen. Med.*, pp. 1–7, Jun. 2023, doi: 10.31487/J.EJGM.2023.01.01.

13. D. T. Burrow, J. T. Heggestad, D. S. Kinnamon, and A. Chilkoti, "Engineering Innovative Interfaces for Point-of-Care Diagnostics," *Curr. Opin. Colloid Interface Sci.*, vol. 66, p. 101718, Jun. 2023, doi: 10.1016/J.COCIS.2023.101718.
14. Q. Liu, X. Jin, J. Cheng, H. Zhou, Y. Zhang, and Y. Dai, "Advances in the Application of Molecular Diagnostic Techniques for the Detection of Infectious Disease Pathogens (Review)," *Mol. Med. Rep.*, vol. 27, no. 5, May 2023, doi: 10.3892/MMR.2023.12991.
15. L. S. Eberlin, "Disease Detection and Diagnostics: Multidisciplinary Approaches to Address Medical Challenges," *JACS Au*, vol. 3, no. 5, pp. 1264–1266, May 2023, doi: 10.1021/JACSAU.3C00196.
16. I. A. Quintela, T. Vasse, C. S. Lin, and V. C. H. Wu, "Advances, Applications, and Limitations of Portable and Rapid Detection Technologies for Routinely Encountered Foodborne Pathogens," *Front. Microbiol.*, vol. 13, Dec. 2022, doi: 10.3389/FMICB.2022.1054782.
17. H. Labinsky et al., "Pos1202-HPR Addressing axSpA Diagnostic Delay by Implementation of Asynchronous Telemedicine and Medical Student-Supported Visits," *Ann. Rheum. Dis.*, vol. 82, no. Suppl 1, pp. 933–934, May 2023, doi: 10.1136/ANNRHEUMDIS-2023-EULAR.2059.
18. K. Papageorgiou and G. Papageorgiou, "An Innovative Method and a Medical Screening Device for Cancer Detection in Real-Time," *Ann. Math. Phys.*, vol. 6, no. 1, pp. 075–082, Jun. 2023, doi: 10.17352/AMP.000084.
19. J. F. Lopez and R. J. Bryant, "The 'Rapid Access Prostate Imaging and Diagnosis' (RAPID) Diagnostic Pathway: What Is the Rush?" *BJUI Int.*, vol. 131, no. 4, pp. 377–379, Feb. 2023, doi: 10.1111/BJU.15971.
20. F. Fuchs et al., "Diagnostic Delay Stages and Pre-Diagnostic Treatment in Patients with Suspected Rheumatic Diseases before Special Care Consultation: Results of a Multicenter-Based Study," *Rheumatol. Int.*, vol. 43, no. 3, pp. 495–502, Oct. 2022, doi: 10.1007/S00296-022-05223-Z.
21. E. Gülçek, M. Yalçinsoy, İ. Gülçek, A. Nakiş Güven, H. Ermiş, and Z. A. Aytemur, "Delays in Diagnosis and Treatment in Patients Underwent Endobronchial Ultrasound-Transbronchial Needle Aspiration (EBUS-TBNA)," *Int. J. Clin. Pract.*, vol. 2022, pp. 1–6, Jul. 2022, doi: 10.1155/2022/7546012.
22. T. V. Nguyen et al., "Efficient Automated Error Detection in Medical Data Using Deep-Learning and Label-Clustering," *Sci. Rep.*, vol. 13, no. 1, Mar. 2023, doi: 10.1038/s41598-023-45946-y.
23. M. E. Al Otaybi et al., "The Quality of Medical Test Results Using Techniques," *Int. J. Bio-Med. Inform. e-Health*, vol. 10, no. 6, pp. 59–63, Nov. 2022, doi: 10.30534/IJBMIEH/2022/101062022.
24. H. L. Bhavyashree and G. Varaprasad, "Morbidity Detection from Clinical Text Data Using Artificial Intelligence Technique," *Data Management, Analytics and Innovation. Lect. Notes Networks Syst.*, vol. 662 LNNS, pp. 383–392, Jan. 2023, doi: 10.1007/978-981-99-1414-2_29.
25. M. A. Dakka et al., "Automated Detection of Poor-Quality Data: Case Studies in Healthcare," *Sci. Rep.*, vol. 11, no. 1, p. 18005, Apr. 2021, doi: 10.1038/S41598-021-97341-0.
26. M. S. Naeem et al., "Evaluating the Safety and Quality of Diagnostic Colonoscopies Performed by General Surgeons: A Retrospective Study," *Cureus*, vol. 15, May 2023, doi: 10.7759/CUREUS.38955.
27. W. Latos et al., "Colonoscopy: Preparation and Potential Complications," *Diagnostics*, vol. 12, no. 3, pp. 747, Mar. 2022, doi: 10.3390/DIAGNOSTICS12030747.
28. S. Yang et al., "Procedural Complications Associated with Invasive Diagnostic Procedures after Lung Cancer Screening with Low-Dose Computed Tomography," *Lung Cancer*, vol. 165, pp. 141–144, Jan. 2022, doi: 10.1016/J.LUNGCAN.2021.12.020.

29. H. Zhao, Y. Xu, J. Huo, A. C. Burks, D. E. Ost, and Y. C. T. Shih, "Updated Analysis of Complication Rates Associated with Invasive Diagnostic Procedures after Lung Cancer Screening," *JAMA Netw. Open*, vol. 3, no. 12, Dec. 2020, doi: 10.1001/JAMANETWORKOPEN.2020.29874.
30. M. Elhadary et al., "Applications of Machine Learning in Chronic Myeloid Leukemia," *Diagnostics*, vol. 13, no. 7, p. 1330, Apr. 2023, doi: 10.3390/DIAGNOSTICS13071330.
31. J. Brecht, M. Chung, and R. Pea, "CML—The ClassSync Modeling Language," *Comput. Support Collab. Learn.*, pp. 189–198, Jan. 2023, doi: 10.4324/9781315045467-28.
32. V. Malik, R. Mittal, and A. Rana, "BiCNN-CML: Hybrid Deep Learning Approach for Chronic Myeloid Leukemia," *Proc. 5th Int. Conf. Contemp. Comput. Informatics, IC3I 2022*, pp. 1771–1777, Dec. 2022, doi: 10.1109/IC3I56241.2022.10073460.
33. S. Iqbal, A. N. Qureshi, J. Li, and T. Mahmood, "On the Analyses of Medical Images Using Traditional Machine Learning Techniques and Convolutional Neural Networks," *Arch. Comput. Methods Eng.*, vol. 30, no. 5, pp. 3173–3233, Apr. 2023, doi: 10.1007/S11831-023-09899-9.
34. M. Hassouna, M. Al-Antary, M. Saleh, and N. B. Al Barghuthi, "Applications of Deep Learning in Medical Imaging: A Brief Review," *2023 Adv. Sci. Eng. Technol. Int. Conf. ASET 2023*, pp. 1–4, Feb. 2023, doi: 10.1109/ASET56582.2023.10180645.
35. T. J. Haight and A. Eshaghi, "Deep Learning Algorithms for Brain Imaging," *Neurology*, vol. 100, no. 12, pp. 549–550, Jan. 2023, doi: 10.1212/WNL.0000000000206808.
36. A. Shrivastava, M. Chakkaravathy, and M. A. Shah, "A Comprehensive Analysis of Machine Learning Techniques in Biomedical Image Processing Using Convolutional Neural Network," *Proc. 5th Int. Conf. Contemp. Comput. Informatics, IC3I 2022*, pp. 1363–1369, Dec. 2022, doi: 10.1109/IC3I56241.2022.10072911.
37. I. Bolodurina, A. Shukhman, L. Legashev, L. Grishina, and A. Zhigalov, "Extracting and Processing of Russian Unstructured Clinical Texts for a Medical Decision Support System," *Eng. Proc.*, vol. 33, no. 1, pp. 14–16, Jun. 2023, doi: 10.3390/ENGPROC2023033041.
38. S. S. Patil and V. Moorthy, "Extraction of Unstructured Electronic Healthcare Records Using Natural Language Processing," *Proc. 1st IEEE Int. Conf. Netw. Commun. 2023, ICNWC 2023,* Apr. 2023, doi: 10.1109/ICNWC57852.2023.10127351.
39. S. Agrawal et al., "Development of Natural Language Processing (NLP) Models for Extracting Key Features from Unstructured Notes to Create Real-World Data (RWD) Assets for Clinical Research at Scale," *J. Clin. Oncol.*, vol. 41, no. 16_suppl, p. 6607, Jun. 2023, doi: 10.1200/JCO.2023.41.16_SUPPL.6607.
40. K. Poudel, M. Uddin, R. Kommu, S. Muhammed, N. Hasan, and S. Hamdan, "HealthCare Text Analytics Using Recent ML Techniques," *Proceedings of the 2023 International Conference on Advances in Computing Research (ACR'23). Lect. Notes Networks Syst.*, vol. 700 LNNS, pp. 134–142, Jan. 2023, doi: 10.1007/978-3-031-33743-7_11.
41. P. Sanchez, J. P. Voisey, T. Xia, H. I. Watson, A. Q. O'Neil, and S. A. Tsaftaris, "Causal Machine Learning for Healthcare and Precision Medicine," *R. Soc. Open Sci.*, vol. 9, no. 8, May 2022, doi: 10.1098/RSOS.220638.
42. F. Scipione, K. Gibbs, and C. Verini, "CML-446 Unfiltered Patient Insights: Commonalities and Differences in Living with Chronic Myeloid Leukemia and Multiple Myeloma," *Clin. Lymphoma. Myeloma Leuk.*, vol. 22, no. Suppl 2, pp. S299–S300, Oct. 2022, doi: 10.1016/S2152-2650(22)01387-8.
43. S. Scholz et al., "Listen to the Patients! Identifying CML Patients' Needs Using AI-Driven Methodologies (Preprint)," JMIR Preprint, Nov. 2022, doi: 10.2196/PREPRINTS.44716.
44. "Cognitive Machine Learning System." Sep. 29, 2015. Accessed: Jun. 08, 2024. [Online]. Available: https://typeset.io/papers/cognitive-machine-learning-system-3q9boy8839

45. K. H. Hohman et al., "Leveraging Electronic Health Record Data for Timely Chronic Disease Surveillance: The Multi-State EHR-Based Network for Disease Surveillance," *J. Public Heal. Manag. Pract.*, vol. 292, no. 2, pp. 162–173, Mar. 2023, doi: 10.1097/PHH.0000000000001693.
46. K. Azarudeen, S. H. Kumar, T. V. Aswin Vijay, P. Thirukumaran, and V. S. B. Balaji, "Intrusion Detection System Based on Pattern Recognition Using CNN," *Int. Conf. Sustain. Comput. Smart Syst. ICSCSS 2023- Proc.,* pp. 567–574, Jun. 2023, doi: 10.1109/ICSCSS57650.2023.10169670.
47. D. V. Jeyanthi and B. Indrani, "IoT-Based Intrusion Detection System for Healthcare Using RNNBiLSTM Deep Learning Strategy with Custom Features," *Soft Comput.*, vol. 27, no. 16, pp. 11915–11930, May 2023, doi: 10.1007/S00500-023-08536-8.
48. S. H. A. Shah, S. Mumtaz, and W. Wei, "Introduction to the Special Issue on Cognitive Computing for Internet of Medical Things in Smart Healthcare," *ACM Trans. Sens. Netw.*, vol. 19, no. 3, pp. 1–3, Apr. 2023, doi: 10.1145/3584742.
49. P. Dini, A. Elhanashi, A. Begni, S. Saponara, Q. Zheng, and K. Gasmi, "Overview on Intrusion Detection Systems Design Exploiting Machine Learning for Networking Cybersecurity," *Appl. Sci.*, vol. 13, no. 13, p. 7507, Jun. 2023, doi: 10.3390/APP13137507.
50. J. Rumbut, H. Fang, S. Carreiro, D. Smelson, and E. Boyer, "An Overview of Wearable Biosensor Systems for Real-Time Substance Use Detection," *IEEE Internet Things J.*, vol. 9, no. 23, pp. 23405–23415, Dec. 2022, doi: 10.1109/JIOT.2022.3207090.
51. A. A. Smith, R. Li, and Z. T. H. Tse, "Reshaping Healthcare with Wearable Biosensors," *Sci. Rep.*, vol. 13, no. 1, Mar. 2023, doi: 10.1038/S41598-022-26951-Z.
52. J. R. Sempionatto, J. A. Lasalde-Ramírez, K. Mahato, J. Wang, and W. Gao, "Wearable Chemical Sensors for Biomarker Discovery in the Omics Era," *Nat. Rev. Chem.*, vol. 6, no. 12, pp. 899–915, Nov. 2022, doi: 10.1038/S41570-022-00439-W.
53. R. Guetari, H. Ayari, and H. Sakly, "Computer-Aided Diagnosis Systems: A Comparative Study of Classical Machine Learning versus Deep Learning-Based Approaches," *Knowl. Inf. Syst.*, vol. 65, no. 10, pp. 1–41, May 2023, doi: 10.1007/S10115-023-01894-7.
54. S. S. Prakash, K. Harshitha, A. O. Charitha, C. Janvitha, and K. Indu, "Computer-Aided Diagnosis using Machine Learning Techniques," *Proc. -2023 3rd Int. Conf. Smart Data Intell. ICSMDI 2023,* pp. 387–391, Mar. 2023, doi: 10.1109/ICSMDI57622.2023.00075.
55. K. A. S. Davis, M. Broadbent, D. Bishara, C. Mueller, and R. Stewart, "Can Medication Mentions in Electronic Health Record Databases Be Used for Researching Medication Use in Older People with Dementia? Comparing the Output of the CRIS Natural Language Processing App for Medicines to GP Prescribing," *medRxiv*, Jan. 2023, doi: 10.1101/2023.01.27.23285104.
56. J. Staal et al., "Effect on Diagnostic Accuracy of Cognitive Reasoning Tools for the Workplace Setting: Systematic Review and Meta-Analysis," *BMJ Qual. Saf.*, vol. 31, no. 12, pp. 899–910, Sep. 2022, doi: 10.1136/BMJQS-2022-014865.
57. A. R. S. V. G. Zhang, "Enhancing Tabular Reasoning with Pattern Exploiting Training," *2nd Conf. Asia-Pacific Chap. Assoc. Comput. Linguist. 12th Int. Joint Conf. Nat. Lang. Process.,* Oct. 2022, pp. 706–726. doi: 10.48550/ARXIV.2210.12259.
58. A. Carpio, A. Simón, A. Torres, and L. F. Villa, "Pattern Recognition in Data as a Diagnosis Tool," *J. Math. Ind.*, vol. 12, no. 1, pp. 1–24, Jan. 2022, doi: 10.1186/S13362-022-00119-W.
59. C. Bu et al., "Cognitive Diagnostic Model Made More Practical by Genetic Algorithm," *IEEE Trans. Emerg. Top. Comput. Intell.*, vol. 7, no. 2, pp. 447–461, Apr. 2023, doi: 10.1109/TETCI.2022.3182692.
60. P. Croskerry, S. G. Campbell, and D. A. Petrie, "The Challenge of Cognitive Science for Medical Diagnosis," *Cogn. Res. Princ. Implic.*, vol. 8, no. 1, Feb. 2023, doi: 10.1186/S41235-022-00460-Z.

61. S. Patel, "An Overview and Application of Deep Convolutional Neural Networks for Medical Image Segmentation," *Proc. 3rd Int. Conf. Artif. Intell. Smart Energy, ICAIS 2023*, pp. 722–728, Feb. 2023, doi: 10.1109/ICAIS56108.2023.10073857.
62. S. Prasher, L. Nelson, and A. Sharma, "Evaluation of Convolution Neural Network Models Using Clinical Datasets," *Emerging Trends in Expert Applications and Security. Lect. Notes Networks Syst.*, vol. 682 LNNS, pp. 253–265, Jan. 2023, doi: 10.1007/978-981-99-1946-8_23.
63. J. Kenei and E. Opiyo, "Modeling and Visualization of Clinical Texts to Enhance Meaningful and User-Friendly Information Retrieval," *2nd Int. Electron. Conf. Healthc.*, Feb. 2023, p. 9. doi: 10.3390/iech2022-12294.
64. O. T. Aduragba, J. Yu, A. Cristea, and Y. Long, "Improving Health Mention Classification Through Emphasising Literal Meanings: A Study Towards Diversity and Generalisation for Public Health Surveillance," *ACM Web Conf. 2023- Proc. World Wide Web Conf. WWW 2023*, vol. 23, pp. 3928–3936, Apr. 2023, doi: 10.1145/3543507.3583877.
65. T. Botsis and K. Kreimeyer, "Improving Drug Safety with Adverse Event Detection Using Natural Language Processing," *Expert Opin. Drug Saf.*, vol. 22, no. 8, pp. 659–668, Jun. 2023, doi: 10.1080/14740338.2023.2228197.
66. A. Chen, Z. Yu, X. Yang, Y. Guo, J. Bian, and Y. Wu, "Contextualized Medication Information Extraction Using Transformer-Based Deep Learning Architectures," *J. Biomed. Inform.*, vol. 142, Mar. 2023, doi: 10.1016/j.jbi.2023.104370.
67. R. Sousa, J. Machado, C. Rodrigues, and L. M. Gomes, "Drug-Drug Interaction Extraction-Based System: An NLP Approach," *Authorea Prepr.*, Mar. 2023, doi: 10.22541/AU.167766849.91957820/V1.
68. A. H. Khatri, V. Gadag, S. Singh, S. K. Satapathy, and S. Mishra, "Quantum Data Traffic Analysis for Intrusion Detection System," *Evol. Appl. Quantum Comput.*, pp. 125–143, May 2023, doi: 10.1002/9781119905172.CH8.
69. C. Chakraborty, S. M. Nagarajan, G. G. Devarajan, T. V. Ramana, and R. Mohanty, "Intelligent AI-Based Healthcare Cyber Security System Using Multi-Source Transfer Learning Method," *ACM Trans. Sens. Netw.*, May 2023, doi: 10.1145/3597210.
70. L. Xie, Y. Ouyang, L. Chen, Z. Wu, and Q. Li, "Towards Better Modeling with Missing Data: A Contrastive Learning-Based Visual Analytics Perspective," *IEEE Trans. Vis. Comput. Graph.*, pp. 1–18, Jan. 2023, doi: 10.1109/TVCG.2023.3285210.
71. S. Dai and D. Svetina Valdivia, "Dealing with Missing Responses in Cognitive Diagnostic Modeling," *Psych*, vol. 4, no. 2, pp. 318–342, Jun. 2022, doi: 10.3390/psych4020028.
72. A. R. Ugale and A. D. Potgantwar, "Anomaly Based Intrusion Detection through Efficient Machine Learning Model," *Int. J. Electr. Electron. Res.*, vol. 11, no. 2, pp. 616–622, Jun. 2023, doi: 10.37391/IJEER.110251.
73. P. U. Eze, N. Geard, I. Mueller, and I. Chades, "Anomaly Detection in Endemic Disease Surveillance Data Using Machine Learning Techniques," *Healthcare*, vol. 11, no. 13, May 2023, doi: 10.3390/healthcare11131896.
74. M. A. Cifci, S. Hussain, and P. J. Canatalay, "Hybrid Deep Learning Approach for Accurate Tumor Detection in Medical Imaging Data," *Diagnostics*, vol. 13, no. 6, p. 1025, Mar. 2023, doi: 10.3390/DIAGNOSTICS13061025.
75. J. D. Rose, R. Vinston Raja, D. Lakshmi, S. Saranya, and T. A. Mohanaprakash, "Privacy Preserving and Time Series Analysis of Medical Dataset Using Deep Feature Selection," *Int. J. Recent Innov. Trends Comput. Commun.*, vol. 11, no. 3, pp. 51–57, Apr. 2023, doi: 10.17762/IJRITCC.V11I3.6201.
76. P. Malik and S. Singh, "Deep Learning Approaches and Biomarkers in Medical Diagnosis," *Recent Patents Eng.*, vol. 17, no. 3, pp. 13–26, Jan. 2023, doi: 10.2174/1872212117666230130100048.

77. T. Sukumar, V. Vidhya, S. Aiswarya, S. Nagavignesh, and J. Hariharan, "Penta Cancer Detection Using Deep Learning Technique," *Adv. Intell. Syst. Comput.*, pp. 781–796, Jan. 2023, doi: 10.1007/978-981-19-9819-5_56.
78. G. Nassreddine, J. Younis, and T. Falahi, "Detecting Data Outliers with Machine Learning," *Al-Salam J. Eng. Technol.*, vol. 2, no. 2, pp. 152–164, May 2023, doi: 10.55145/AJEST.2023.02.02.018.
79. M. Kumar, S. A. Khan, A. Bhatia, V. Sharma, and P. Jain, "A Conceptual Introduction of Machine Learning Algorithms," *2023 1st Int. Conf. Intell. Comput. Res. Trends, ICRT 2023*, pp. 1–7, Feb. 2023, doi: 10.1109/ICRT57042.2023.10146676.
80. D. Samariya, J. Ma, S. Aryal, and X. Zhao, "Detection and Explanation of Anomalies in Healthcare Data," *Health. Inf. Sci. Syst.*, vol. 11, no. 1, Apr. 2023, doi: 10.1007/S13755-023-00221-2.
81. T. Lohanan et al., "Development and Validation of a Screening Instrument for Borderline Personality Disorder (SI-Bord) for Use Among University Students," *BMC Psychiatry*, vol. 20, no. 1, Aug. 2020, doi: 10.1186/S12888-020-02807-6.
82. I. O. Muraina, M. A. Agoi, B. O. Omorojor, A. A. Adedokun, and R. O. Ajetunmobi, "Decision Making and Machine Learning Algorithms' Selection with Artificial Intelligent Rule-Based Expert System," *Int. J. Res. Sci. Innov.*, vol. 09, no. 04, pp. 54–60, 2022, doi: 10.51244/IJRSI.2022.9406.
83. T. Grote and P. Berens, "Uncertainty, Evidence, and the Integration of Machine Learning into Medical Practice.," *J. Med. Philos.*, vol. 48, no. 1, pp. 84–97, Jan. 2023, doi: 10.1093/JMP/JHAC034.
84. A. Fansi Tchango, R. Goel, J. Martel, Z. Wen, G. Marceau Caron, and J. Ghosn, "Towards Trustworthy Automatic Diagnosis Systems by Emulating Doctors' Reasoning with Deep Reinforcement Learning," *Adv. Neural Inf. Process. Syst.,* 2022, vol. 35, pp. 24502–24515. [Online]. Available: https://proceedings.neurips.cc/paper_files/paper/2022/file/9b6c8c4a5aeb6a37c9efa963e30993d9-Paper-Conference.pdf
84. S. W. Betsy, A. Murugesan, N. B. S. Ganapathy, and N. Pughazendi, "A Novel Framework for Network Intrusion Detection in Healthcare Domain," *ICSPC 2023–4th Int. Conf. Signal Process. Commun.,* pp. 43–46, Mar. 2023, doi: 10.1109/ICSPC57692.2023.10125636.
86. H. Kaur and A. Malik, "Review on Cognitive Computing Techniques in Healthcare," *ICSCCC 2023-3rd Int. Conf. Secur. Cyber Comput. Commun.*, pp. 536–541, May 2023, doi: 10.1109/ICSCCC58608.2023.10176762.
87. S. Rangaraju, "Secure by Intelligence: Enhancing Products with AI-Driven Security Measures," *EPH - Int. J. Sci. Eng.*, vol. 9, no. 3, pp. 36–41, Dec. 2023, doi: 10.53555/EPHIJSE.V9I3.212.
88. P. Gupta and D. D. Seth, "Early Detection of Heart Disease Using Multilayer Perceptron," *Micro-Electronics and Telecommunication Engineering. Lect. Notes Networks Syst.*, vol. 617 LNNS, pp. 309–315, Jun. 2023, doi: 10.1007/978-981-19-9512-5_28.
89. W. Y. Tan, C. Hargreaves, C. Chen, and S. Hilal, "A Machine Learning Approach for Early Diagnosis of Cognitive Impairment Using Population-Based Data," *J. Alzheimer's Dis.*, vol. 91, no. 1, pp. 449–461, Jan. 2023, doi: 10.3233/JAD-220776.
90. M. Fabietti et al., "Early Detection of Alzheimer's Disease from Cortical and Hippocampal Local Field Potentials Using an Ensembled Machine Learning Model," *IEEE Trans. Neural Syst. Rehabil. Eng.*, vol. 31, pp. 2839–2848, Jun. 2023, doi: 10.1109/TNSRE.2023.3288835.
91. R. A. Rayan, "Machine Learning for Smart Health Care," *Mach. Learn. Algorithms Appl. Eng.*, pp. 1–16, Jan. 2023, doi: 10.1201/9781003104858-1.

Index

For Product Safety Concerns and Information please contact our EU
representative GPSR@taylorandfrancis.com
Taylor & Francis Verlag GmbH, Kaufingerstraße 24, 80331 München, Germany

www.ingramcontent.com/pod-product-compliance
Ingram Content Group UK Ltd.
Pitfield, Milton Keynes, MK11 3LW, UK
UKHW021826101126
477531UK00019B/411
9781032745701